'SICK & TIRED OF BEING SICK & TIRED':

Solutions for a Better, Healthier Life

Table Of Contents

1
OVERVIEW

I'm sick & tired of:

1. **America being obese & overweight (as a kid growing up 15 people could fit in an elevator, now only 3).**

2. *my friends & family dying way too young.*

3. **people coming to me injured, sick & out of shape to tell me everything they know about health.**

4. *lazy, out-of-touch doctors who would rather write a prescription than offer sound guidance on how to eat and exercise.*

5. **the fitness industry preying on people who need real help.**

6. *hearing people blame their genetics for their health woes when the truth is that it's their lifestyle.*

7. **finicky eaters of all ages.**

8. *how physically weak America has become.*

9. **erectile dysfunction commercials.**

10. *people who tell me how many steps they took today.*

11. **20 year old fitness gurus.**

12. *those who tell me how their doctor told them how fit they are but that they have to stay on 3 LifeTime medications.*

13. **the 2 major obstacles to everyone's health... misinformation & habits.**

14. *health experts who either look anything but healthy or are on a PED needle (performance enhancing drugs).*

15. **yoga classes filled with uncontrollable gas. If all the world became vegetarians, it would be people emitting vast quantities of methane gas replacing cows as #1.**

16. *everyone being braced- ankles, knees, backs, elbows, wrists, necks. Braces can hold you up BUT eventually they hold you back.*

17. **of desperate people signing up for the 'quick fix'- gastric bypass, gastric sleeves, vitamins, magic potions and 'lose weight quick' scams.**

18. *people being tired with no energy or vitality & not knowing what to do about it.*

19. **hearing how people can't get a deep sleep without drugs.** Note: sleep is as important as diet and exercise.

20. *folks not being able to 'live the life' they desperately want to live.*

21. **hearing people complain of back & neck pain with their only solution being drugs.**

22. *folks wasting money on bogus exercise equipment.*

23. **the food industry and how government approves of health-killing 'foods' to eat (follow the money).**

24. *the fight-cancer industry(follow the money)*

25. **parents & grandparents unable to participate in energetic activities with their families.**

26. people thinking it's normal to be abnormal and saying 'it's just the way I am'.

I try not to offend anyone. But if I do, it's with Love in my Heart.

Why my Job is so Difficult- Dealing with people who are so smart and experienced regarding their personal health and wellness doesn't allow them to hear my voice. Yet, these same people are sick, overweight, weak, injured, taking meds and generally feel awful.

Compared to what everyone accepts as a 'healthy' way to live, my system is radical. Yet once learned and understood, it's quite simple & 'doable' but radical in today's accepted ways. Feeling is understanding.

How can my small voice compete with the sculpted young experts of our time? These young brash Health & Fitness experts were expounding their wisdom when I was young as well. But most all have disappeared since the needle they were on betrayed them. Their shortcuts did not stand the test of time. But so many people poured out their sweat and hard earned money on the promise of a beautiful, healthy, pain-free body.

The gimmicks of those selling fitness have not changed much in the last 100 years.

So why listen to this voice? 65 years on this planet has taught me a few things. But what I know as true is not just theory or from a certification class or from an infomercial full of experts. Or even from the plain old youthful exuberance of believing that the way they train themselves is effective for all who 'buy in'. Heck in my 20s I could live on beer, pizza and ice cream and STILL have great abs!

But what are you going to do on that day when the cumulative effect of all your deleterious exercises and misguided eating and poorly informed way of supplementing catches up? One of my favorite words is 'cumulative'. In this case, it could take years to undo all the bad stuff. It's like you have to develop a new 'cumulative'. But it's not like you just have to change the way you train or eat or supplement and all is well.

It won't be that easy. The hardest part is changing your mind. But you must because this is really important. It's your health, your very life!

I'm so glad I learned this stuff. I'm glad I was humble enough to seek out great teachers and mentors. Well actually I was forced to be humble. All my injuries were crippling. But I still had hope and that allowed me to start over. And now I'm in better shape than I was 25 years ago and I exercise less than 2 hours a week!

I would love to help guide you through all the nonsense. Let's talk. Honest talk, honest results.

65 can be the next 40 for you! Extend the middle years!

Old maxim- 5 words> eat less and exercise more

New maxim- 5 words> eat smart and exercise smarter

I am 65 so my experience is just that- experience... and not theory. Not only can I share with you what works; I can actually demonstrate the strength in all of us.

Learn & Adopt Vital Lifestyle Habits That Will Greatly Lower the Need for 'Sick' Care!

Minimal Exercise with Maximal Focus yields the Greatest Benefit!

And this is why what I'm proposing is DIFFERENT than anything else out there---

If you need to:

- ❖ **Lose Weight, Get Off Lifetime Medications & OTC Drugs**

- ❖ **Overcome Injuries, Get Stronger, Learn How to Train YOUR particular Body**

- ❖ **Sleep Better Without Drugs**

- ❖ **Set Realistic Goals & Reach Them**

❖ **Have Great Blood/Lab Reports for Lower Health & Life Insurance Rates**

THE word is **CUMULATIVE**!

Defined as:

⇒ *increasing or becoming better or worse over time through a series of additions*

⇒ *including or adding together all of the things that came before*

When we truly grasp the meaning of this word, life changes for the better!

Too much of how we eat & exercise is based on wrong or inaccurate assumptions that SEEM to make sense.

❖ The National Center for Health Statistics reports that low back pain accounts for 13 million visits to doctors each year, with 14.3% of all new doctor visits attributed to lower back pain; it is also the most frequent reason given for lost productivity in the USA.

❖ Also 66% of all American adults are taking Prescription Drugs and the number is 75% for us over 50. Pause & think about that especially since ALL drugs have side effects.

I don't think people <u>really</u> understand how easy a Healthy Lifestyle can truly be. Instead of telling folks to 'eat healthy' (whatever that means) or to 'get some exercise' (whatever that means), I look at the 'complete' person.

Stress Kills and Speeds up Aging---

Genetics loads the gun; Lifestyle pulls the Trigger!

2

THE BEGINNING

The Beginning- Sickly Kid whose Mom took control

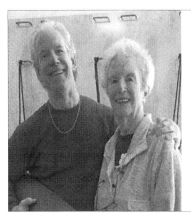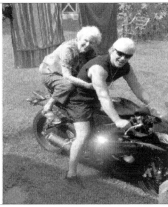

This is about my education and real life experiences that might qualify me to speak about health and fitness. Although I have formal training by way of physical education type courses as well as Anatomy & Physiology, Applied Kinesiology and General Nutrition and professional certifications, it's the real-life laboratory experiences that have had the most profound effect. By this I mean that my education goes way beyond the classroom. In fact it began before I was even old enough to go to kindergarten.

As all parents know, things don't always work according to plan and I was not the healthiest of kids. In fact, I almost died at the age of four during one of my tougher bouts with bronchial asthma. This event really got Mom's attention.

My Mom joined forces with some of the original 'health nuts'. She wanted her new baby boy to be in perfect health and never get hurt and never cry and be very smart and handsome and happy. To this end, Mom jumped on board with health pioneers like Adelle Davis, Carlton Fredricks, Gaylord Hauser, and the guy on our black & white TV with his dog Happy… none other than Jack LaLanne.

Her diligence helped her uncover all kinds of ways to naturally support my immune system and minimize my dependence on pharmaceuticals. By high school, she even had a year-round system in place that kept me from wheezing every time I exerted myself and from catching every cold, sore throat, flu and other disease that came near me.

So from the very beginning the lab rat was… me. Brewer's yeast, cod liver oil, calf's liver once a week, lecithin, vitamins A, B-complex, C, D, E, calcium, magnesium, other minerals,

Tiger's Milk, fresh fruit and veggies were staples when I was a kid. And never white bread. It was peanut butter and jelly on Whole Wheat bread or cream cheese and walnuts on raisin bread.

One of the best lessons I learned was that eating is not just supposed to be about pleasure for the palate. I learned that food is fuel and nourishment. And when used correctly, can contribute greatly to one's life force.

Over the years, I've made some adjustments to Mom's system. The crazy thing is, that at age 52, I was healthier and physically stronger than I'd been in my entire life. And I'm still going very strong at 65!

Lest you think that my only physical challenge was some bronchial asthma, let me tell you a bit more. There was a period of years when I did not take care of myself and ignored Mom's wisdom. This resulted in mind-numbing headaches (from allergies), a displaced vertebrae in my neck thanks to a hit in football, no cartilage in my right knee from a 'me-being-out-of-shape' basketball injury, alcohol and drug dependency issues. Add to that a motorcycle crash that shattered my left elbow & severed my tricep, tore a hole in my right shin that measured 6x12 inches, ripped up my left knee that took multiple surgeries & spare parts from a cadaver to repair. In

11

addition, I've had a series of low back injuries that from time to time have left me incapacitated, a hiatal hernia, a displaced knuckle on my left hand, rosacea, a skin condition on my right foot, problems with bicep tendonitis in my right rotator cuff, acne, and very high cholesterol (probably a combination of genetics and an inability to properly deal with stress). Oh and a busted up hip from a 20 foot fall with a running chain saw in my hand. But the Tree Story is quite famous now and a great source of encouragement for many.

I've probably left something out but you get the picture. And I'm not complaining since it's good to be alive. The knowledge gained by living through this stuff gives me a perspective that goes beyond a formal classroom or lab. The good news is that I'm loved & excited about every day I am given. It's really hard to believe how incredible the human body is and how it can comeback from near-death injuries and sickness.

If I could overcome all the health problems and go on to be a world-class strongman at my age, I know that you can get on track to reach your health and fitness goals as well. I've also been asked to address the issue of training around and through injuries. No problem.

❖ Growing up in New Jersey in the 1950s... We swam in a mercury- laden river along with other toxic waste, we ran in the cloud behind DDT Spraying trucks in our neighborhoods that was for killing mosquitoes, our walls were painted with Lead paint, our buildings were insulated with Asbestos, factories billowed all kinds of smoke over us, there were no Emission standards for gasoline and diesel cars & trucks, we had only 3 different types of vegetables in our house (ever), I only remember 3 different kinds of fruit, we had no idea of the 'source' of our meats, poultry and fish. Tobacco was allowed just about everywhere except Church and school.

I had measles, German measles, mumps, chicken pox, various flus & asthma when I was a kid. Today I feel fantastic. Bed rest, aspirin, Vick's VapoRub & Calamine lotion were used for everything except for the asthma- they put me in an oxygen tent for a few days when it was really bad. Then my Mom gave up on traditional medicine when they said I was allergic to everything they injected into my arm and they wanted us to get rid of my dog, carpeting, as well as wrap my mattress & pillow in plastic (see BubbleBoy).

Mom said No to just about every Drug along with Inhalers & we kept our dog. The Medical/Science/Pharmaceutical industries are as corrupt as Governments-- sadly follow the money... Current Drug regimens & Immunizations DO NOT Strengthen Immune Systems! (Actually just the opposite seems to occur)

Methinks that the current approach to fighting disease is backwards. The Human Body is nothing less than a Miraculous Gift that has incredible capacities to heal. Instead of dumping tons of resources into 'finding cures' in a laboratory, we would be much better served by getting our planet in order- land, water & air. The earth abounds with cures for 'what ails ya'.

Instead of 'science' being so arrogant in thinking they can improve what is naturally provided in this world, the goal should be to return it to its natural state. Of course that would take a Moral Compass which Governments, many Businesses, Educational Institutions, the Medical Community, the Science Community, the Agricultural Community, and Wall Street have not come close to displaying.

It's a shame because no one gets out alive anyway. And to think we have the God-given tools to greatly decrease Human Suffering yet many would sell their very souls for personal profit at the expense of all humanity. A sad state indeed.

Hoping we can all 'fight the good fight' on all levels with an eye to saving the planet for all generations to follow. I trust there is a Better Life after this!

Some of my other life lessons might help you understand better why so many athletes let themselves physically fall apart when their sport's career ends.

For me personally the high point of my sport's experience was in 9th grade at 15 years old! In the Jersey City, New Jersey basketball championship game against future Hall of Fame Coach Bob Hurley Sr.'s St. Anthony's High School team, I scored 36 points and my team won the 1st championship in school history. The newspaper headline called me the 'Guiding Light'. That term became the name of a soap opera! Too funny. Since I played football and baseball as well, I was voted Athlete of the Year in my town. Well at least I had a high point, right? I'm thankful for that.

But then the environment surrounding the late 1960s got the better of me. Sex, drugs and rock & roll sounded so good but it destroyed my athletic potential as well as other aspects of life. I blew so many opportunities for greatness but I won't bore you with the details.

By the time I turned 21 what I saw in the mirror scared me. It had to be Change or Die. I started by lifting 2 dumbbells at night while watching the Johnny Carson Show from 1130pm until 1am every night. I was going to school full time days then working a full time job in the evenings. I had never lifted weights before so I just made things up to do. The guy who had loaned me the 2 dumbbells would regale me with stories of a famous bodybuilder from my town who had worked the same job as me. Yet now he was Mr. Universe and starring in the movies.

I picked up some bodybuilding magazines and started to picture a healthy body for myself. Not desiring to actually be a bodybuilder, I was just captivated by the idea that the human body could change so dramatically. And I desperately needed change.

Somehow I mustered up the discipline to stop drinking as well as the other things that went with it. My friends thought I had run off and joined a monastery or the French Foreign Legion. I cleaned up my diet but looking back my definition of 'clean' has changed a lot over the years.

After a few months of sitting home at night with the 2 dumbbells, my Dad connected me with one of his clients who owned a hardcore bodybuilding gym in Jersey City, New

Jersey. Actually, many of the guys I had seen in magazines trained there when they were in the NYC area. I used to tune up the owner's motorcycle in exchange for a gym membership.

Early in the morning I would trudge up the long flight of purple stairs to catch a workout before school. Not having the money to pay for the trainer on staff, I just tried to imitate what I saw others do or things I had gleaned from magazines. Leg day was particularly brutal and I would have to slide down the stairs on my butt so that I wouldn't fall head over heels with my wobbly legs.

Unbeknownst to me, many of the guys were shooting up with Dianabol- one of the early anabolic steroids. I could never figure why my progress seemed so slow when others would grow muscles seemingly overnight! But I am so thankful today that I didn't get caught up in that scene. The overall deleterious effects on one's health are just not worth it.

By the end of 18 months my swollen pot belly had disappeared and my arms had grown from a waif-like 11"s up to just about 16"s. I felt stronger and healthier then I had ever been.

It seems like we humans have a propensity to take giant steps forward and then congratulate ourselves so much that we end up taking a few steps back. And that still happens to me. But the good news is that I had started to build a very solid foundation of strength and health that would serve me well in the years to follow.

The big motorcycle crash of '79 is a great example of how being in shape can save your life and then help you recover faster than most. After having 3 limbs surgically repaired and being on my back for 30 days, I was able to hop out of the hospital after only the 2nd day standing up. The doctor had planned on keeping me for at least another month!

A few years later I moved into my first house. Between working full time, trying to run a part-time business and also taking care of my growing family getting my training in was almost impossible. The nearest gym was 10 miles away. But I did have a basement and I decided to put together a home gym. It was pretty basic, nothing fancy and it became known as the Dungeon.

All excuses were eliminated and I regained everything that had been lost. *The great, unanticipated, serendipitous benefit was the example I was setting for my children.* At one point or another they all picked up on what I was doing and why. Over 35 years later, they all are intelligently taking good care of their bodies.

At the ripe old age of 39 my mind was radically opened to the physical possibilities we all have. We had been visiting some friends down at the Jersey shore and they had brought us to hear a famous guitar player perform at their church. During one of the breaks a couple of guys got up and performed some feats of strength. I watched as if I was watching a magician, trying to figure out the trick.

We ended up staying overnight with our friends. My wife had left her purse at the event the night before so the next day we loaded up the kids and went back for the Sunday morn church service. The purse was exactly where she had left it. Thank God it was an honest church!

As I'm sitting on the 2nd row the strongman from the night before was asked to get up and say a few words. He spoke of how he didn't think he was going to be able to make the trip because his 7 year old daughter had died the week before after a long illness.

Having lost a son in a car crash a few years earlier, I immediately flashed back on how real the grieving process was for me. I think we all connect on a deeper level with others who have experienced similar tragic events. After he spoke, the guy sat directly in front of me!

At the conclusion of the service, I reached forward and put my hand on his shoulder. He turned around and I asked if we could talk for a minute, even though I had no clue as to what I was going to say. He started telling me how they had to load up and get on the road because they had a show that night down by Atlantic City. But then all of a sudden he stopped. He briefly spoke to the guy with him then turned back to me and said 'Ok, let's go to lunch'.

We exchanged some wild stories about each of our lives and then he asked if I could help him out. He was feeling pretty sick and needed someone to help break some bricks during the show that night. I thanked him for asking and told him that, basically, I was just an old basketball player. In addition, I wasn't a karate guy and, although I'd lifted some weights, I wasn't particularly strong. He'd better find someone else to do his brick-breaking.

Well, he was insistent and my wife (who's a very supportive woman) said, 'Go ahead and help the guy'. The next thing I knew I was driving down the Garden State Parkway with this guy from San Diego, California and he's telling me about the fine art of breaking bricks. We arrive at the show and there's a big room, packed full of people. There are two large stacks of bricks on the stage and I'm told that the one on the left is mine. Nine 2-inch thick bricks, no practice. Can you picture this?

It was like being at a concert or a sports event. Everyone was pumped. The music was cranking, lights flashing and the crowd was loud. The show starts and I get on stage in front of my stack of bricks. Now, up until this point I was caught up in the excitement. It was great. They started the countdown. 10...9... Suddenly, all of that excitement just drained right out of me. I became filled with fear. This wasn't your ordinary, everyday fear. This was deep, down in your stomach, knees knockin', hands sweatin' when it's cold- FEAR.

I was afraid of three things. First, I was afraid that I was going to break my arm. Second, I was afraid that, once it broke, it was going to be very painful (and I don't like pain). And third, I was afraid that the bricks weren't going to break and everyone was going to be laughing as they took me to the local hospital. It sounds funny now, but it was quite serious at the time.

All of a sudden, right in the middle of the countdown, I remembered part of a speech that I had heard a few years before. The speaker said that faith and fear cannot live in the same body at the same time. I walked around for a week repeating, 'Faith and fear cannot live in the same body at the same time. Faith and fear...' What was this guy talking about?

It finally hit me. He meant that some things in life are all or nothing. It's like your best friend saying to you, 'I'll always be your best friend...99%'. 99%? Wait a minute. How do you know when that 1% is going to sneak in? When will your best friend just leave you?

Either you're my best friend or not. That's it. No in betweens. No almost. Yes or no. All or nothing. It's the same with faith and fear. You choose. What's going to control your life? Look around and see how fear cripples the vast majority of people. Worry, anxiety, panic, doubt, misbelief, mistrust... fear vs. faith, belief, confidence, hope, trust. Which one will you allow to rule your life? Years ago, I read that we are born with two fears- fear of falling and fear of loud noises. All the rest of our fears are learned or imagined. It's definitely something you need to think about as you move ahead with your life.

So anyway, there I was staring at these bricks in a near panic. It was time to put up or shut up. Do or die. I chose total faith, prayed like never before, jumped up, and totally smashed that stack of bricks. They went flying in all directions. There was no one in the place more excited than me. It was wild.

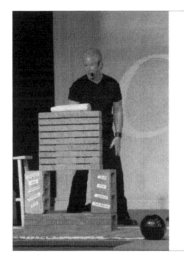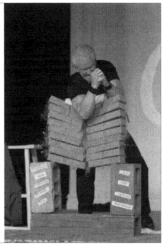

The good news is that you don't have to smash a stack of bricks to break through the wall of negative in your life. The breakthrough actually happened before I even hit the bricks. *The breakthrough came in my mind.* The bricks were just a symbolic detail that forced me to face my fear. You may not have a pile of bricks like I did, but you will have something big that you have to face... and defeat. You may call it a defining moment where, how you respond, will set the course of your life. It will be your test. Know that it's coming. Enjoy it. Choose wisely.

After seeing how doing strength feats that seem almost impossible opened up the audience to whatever message you might want to share, I got excited. At the time I wanted to radically impact young people in a positive way. Strength feats turned out to be my vehicle.

I was fortunate enough to learn from the greatest performing strongman of my generation- Dennis Rogers. It wasn't an easy road though. Dennis doesn't believe in the trickery and illusion that many employ. Everything is real and that meant I had many hours of hard work to get where I needed to be.

The hardest work was to believe.

Now after 27 years and over 1,000 live presentations, the strength is still there but at age 65 the stamina is not what it once was. No worries though. Experience and the wisdom it brings can be a great equalizer!

Today I train differently than years ago. Less is more is so cliché, but compared to how much time the exercise crazies put in, it's me. Around 2 hours of totally focused training a week is the most I put in.

The eating just falls into place, getting it right (by my definition) the vast majority of the time. Listening to my body.

Motivation to get and stay in shape is a funny thing. I vacillate. Vanity versus Health versus Competition. Am I training to just look good? Much of the time 'yes!' So I find it quite amusing when I discover some Sharpei-like skin in different places.

Health motivates me especially seeing many peers succumbing to illness maybe a bit too young. But health also motivates when thinking about extending the active, middle years of my life and also for fast recovery from the injuries we all get from time to time.

Competition is not a big motivator for me personally. I scored enough baskets when I was a kid. But for many competing really gets them fired up. A really intelligent training plan can support the competing athlete. But sadly many do not have the will to do the foundation work and are forced to quit competing much too young.

I'm not an A-type personality so changing my 'sick & tired' paradigm was kind of peaceful... with a comfortable level discipline. Have I mentioned the word 'cumulative' yet? Meditate on that word for a bit.

My Trial & Error Expertise can work for you. My advisor has suggested that I start a community or a tribe or a family or a friendly group of folks who desire to extend the middle years and minimize the damage as we enter our later years and eternity.

3

EXERCISE

The widely-accepted modern American paradigm divides exercise into the 3 areas of Stretching, Cardiovascular Training and Strength Work. Based on my life experiences as well as observations over the years, it is very wrong, incorrect, nonsensical, mistaken, erroneous, unsound, faulty, dangerous and hogwash-ical.

As a nation we have come to accept injuries that require surgery as normal in the course of play or everyday human activity. Seriously? These phenomenally equipped bodies we are born with have been done a disservice. The young people today are dramatically less fit than kids 100 years ago.

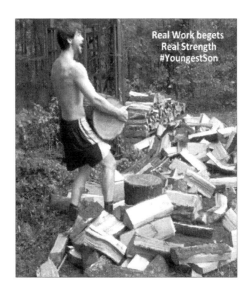

Real Work begets
Real Strength
#YoungestSon

Yet today in our country there seems to be a gymnasium or a yoga studio almost on every corner. Youth sports have greater participation than churches on Sunday mornings. Home exercise equipment abounds & there are walking, jogging and running clubs. We are bombarded with 'scientific studies' about exercise. Also, ads, infomercials and free workout videos abound. And our doctors tell us to exercise more. Heck, here in my home state of New Jersey it is required by law that Physical Therapists have a PhD!

It reminds me of a college visit I went on with one of my children who was being recruited. It was a beautiful campus up in the Northeast. The coach that was showing us around noted how the school was well known as one of the best in the nation for Physical Therapy, Athletic Trainers, Personal Trainers and Dance Exercise.

Most of the student body participate in a sport while doing their under graduate work. They had 2 gigantic gyms with fancy, modern equipment on campus that were available to all. They were full of energetic students that day.

Then he showed us the Trainer's Room which traditionally is used for athletes who are injured or who need to be specially prepared to compete. Oh My Goodness!! The 'room' was bigger than the biggest gym on campus. Rows and rows of tables used to treat the injured. While I was respectful in my reaction when the coach showed it to us, as a parent I felt kind of queasy. All this stuff on campus, all the healthy looking kids, all the activity... *yet injuries were the elephant in the room.*

Have you ever just paused to think why this is the norm in our world today? I have.

Let's do a little test to prove a point. If you can, stand in front of a mirror. Since I love beach muscles, we'll use the bicep. Roll up your sleeve and hoist one elbow up to shoulder height and flex your bicep muscle hard. Now straighten your arm and allow the bicep to totally relax. Got it?

My bicep (as well as the rest of the skeletal muscles in my body) can only do 2 things. They can contract or relax, shorten or lengthen. The one thing they surely don't do is stretch.

So if before, during or after activity you attempt to 'stretch out' a muscle and muscles don't stretch, what are you actually doing? Think about it.

This is a problem since the only things you could be stretching are tendons & ligaments. But tendons & ligaments are supposed to be tight to protect your joints like ankles, knees, hips, back, neck, shoulders, elbows, etc. *And therein you will find one of the greatest problems in the way we teach exercise. We are literally being set up to ... be injured!*

Through some very smart people I've met and learned from, I now know that if I want a greater range of motion, muscles need to relax or turn off. So my training will reflect that. When certain muscles feel very tight and are difficult to relax, I take that as a sign that something is amiss. And if I properly respond to the warning, I will avoid serious injury.

Generally speaking, tight muscles mean that they are in 'protect mode'. The muscles stay partially contracted as a warning that there is an imbalance or weakness somewhere.

Tight hamstrings are classic. People try to stretch the heck out of them and they might feel good when completely warmed up but within an hour of working out, they tighten again. The tight hammies might be protecting a knee or hip or back or they might even be influenced by an old ankle injury that was never properly resolved. Please leave conventional stretching out.

Consider ways to get muscles to contract and relax. You might just find the answer somewhere up the line from your musculoskeletal system. Your tightness could be a neurologic issue or even further up. It could be something in your thought processes like fear.

Just like we talk about a 'holistic' view of medicine. We wouldn't just look at where it hurts unless it's some sort of blunt force trauma or the like. Holistic medicine would consider many factors to come up with a protocol to heal.

The same should be considered when planning exercise. The magnificent human body is designed to have all its parts work in harmony. Every exercise then should be with the entire body in mind. There should be one, unified holistic exercise plan that addresses all of our human systems.

So when speaking about our Physical World-- the key to a healthy life is movement, the key to movement is velocity and the key to velocity is position.

When I am in the right position, contracting the right muscles, relaxing the opposing muscles and am totally mindful as well as intentional during exercise, awesome things occur.

Less Pain, More Function

I would like to give you some 'food for thought' as you embark on a new fitness program or look at the one you have. Since the rage in fitness these days is some derivation of Cross-Fit or High-Intensity Interval Training (HIIT), we should probably look there to see if it's appropriate for you.

By Cross-Training I mean the exercise philosophy that gives one a myriad of different activities to perform in either a given workout session or over the course of days, weeks or months. This would include lifting weights, cardio, and stretching executed in an almost infinite variety of ways.

While 'in theory' this type of training may 'sound good', it might be a wise idea to dig a bit deeper knowing what you know about your personal situation including history of injury. AND you might want to know if these different training programs actually IMPROVE performance- whether you are just looking to function better in your daily activities or are training to be a world class athlete.

Remember that any new activity has a learning curve where one must coordinate oneself to actually do it. Once we learn something new, will it really improve our level of fitness and functionality?

A few years back I was introduced to Jay Schroeder who trains elite-level athletes. His philosophy was much different than anything I had come across in my 1st 25 years in the fitness field. Jay believed that position is of critical importance in training followed by velocity. He challenged me to test his theory.

My youngest son was just finishing 10th grade and was always getting injured in sports. He became the subject of this new training experiment. Wrestling and baseball were his sports and although he had 'skills', he was really lacking in speed and strength.

In June he was tested in the mile run and his time was 6:48. In September he was re-tested. His time dropped to 6:00! He improved by a full 48 seconds and yet he had not run at all the entire summer – not even to the mailbox! He went from last to 2nd in team sprints and he recovered faster than anyone. His workouts were 4 exercises performed 4 days a week for 5 minutes per movement- never lifting a weight, doing any cardio and never stretching. 25 minutes of real work x 4 days per week= 100 minutes total time per week. Under 2 hours a week for 3 months yielded inconceivable results.

My son learned how to activate the right muscles at the right time and by doing so he turned off all opposing muscles. The same way you get faster and stronger is the same way you overcome and recover from injury.

As a college wrestler, one summer he trained in Jay's gym in Arizona. The heaviest weight he trained with over 2 months was 8 lbs and he never ran or stretched yet he came back in the best shape ever in his 21 years on the planet. Since his college coach insists on heavy lifting, my son asked the guys out west how to improve his Bench Press. His best-ever lift had been 3 reps @ 185 lbs which is not very impressive at all. (In his defense, my son has very long limbs and an above normal level of joint laxity so being a great weightlifter would never happen. He did have great success in wrestling however.) After a brief instruction on which muscles to activate and when, he executed 11 perfect form reps @ 185. Then they put 225 on the bar and he did 3 more — never having lifted over 185 in his life!

We are all incredibly strong as humans. If we can only learn to utilize the correct muscles at the proper time and always look to improve our position, we can live lives with less pain and more function than we might dare to believe.

I get it though. You've been led to believe that Cardio and Stretching are right up there with Strength Training to get you in fantastic shape, lose weight and have improved overall health. So why not do the much easier, mindless stuff?

Set the treadmill and the earth spins beneath your feet & you perspire. You can even watch the news or a soap or a game while 'exercising'. But you are doing your body a disservice and wasting your time.

Chronic cardio as it's called has not been living up to its promise. Very few bodies are equipped to even handle the local jog around the neighborhood. A slightly elevated heart rate is of no benefit. Even with fancy running shoes, pounding your joints on a usually uneven street surface is just a series of injuries waiting to happen.

A new string of studies has found evidence of higher arterial plaque levels in the most active endurance athletes. Yes, there is a proclivity toward heart problems found in endurance athletes- atherosclerosis, cardiac arrhythmias, and other heart troubles.

Need proof? Researchers have been doing comparisons between traditional endurance training and more intense forms of exercise like strength training or sprint interval training. Cardio always loses.

What's better for altering body composition—resistance training alone, endurance training alone, or endurance training with resistance training?

Resistance training is always the answer leading to greater fat loss and retention of lean muscle mass while also reducing fasting insulin levels and improving blood lipids.

In obese teens, strength training alone reduced body fat more than endurance training.

What about "unhealthy" people with conditions like heart failure or diabetes? Are they too fragile to endure resistance training? Would an hour long jog be a better, safer use of their time? The answer is no. Jogging through your neighborhood or cycling for three hours just doesn't cover all your bases like a full-body strength workout.

Diabetes researchers examining this exact issue are quick to say that "more exercise is not better" and that it's all in how you exercise. You can't just do something that gets you fatigued and hope you're destroying your glucose intolerance, insulin resistance, and normalizing your glucose levels. You have to train the actual muscles that will be accepting or rejecting the glucose. And the absolute best way is to move those muscles.

As humans, we are not fragile. You were not born a snowflake! *We can tolerate intense exercise or just some hard physical work. Conversely, we cannot tolerate avoiding intense exercise.*

All this should be great news for women in particular. In many respects, you have it harder. You often take on more domestic responsibilities while still working, and yet the conventional wisdom is that you mustn't lift too many weights or damage your delicate bodies with strength training. You want toned muscles not big, bulky ones. And so you end up taking hour-long Pilates classes or doing 45-minute light aerobics sessions or taking a restorative yoga class when you could learn about Intelligent Strength and get better results in minutes, not hours!

If you're getting paid to run marathons or compete in triathlons, keep doing it. You've got the justification you need to tax your body and perform what probably amounts to a suboptimal training regimen. Just be sure to get out while you can still walk and move well.

Get a Grip on Your Health: Can Freaky Forearms Predict How Healthy You Will Be & How Long You Will Live?

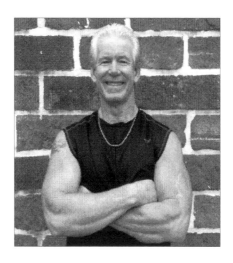

Back in 1992 at the ripe old age of 39 I happened to meet Dennis Rogers. Dennis would go on to become the GrandMaster Strongman of his generation. He didn't look like the hulking behemoths we are accustomed to seeing. Actually at about 5'9" and 149 pounds he appeared quite diminutive. But the adage 'looks can be deceiving' was probably written with Dennis in mind.

A 2-time World Arm Wrestling Champion, his signature strength feat was holding back two US Army training planes at full throttle from taking off. His hand and grip feats are legend. Placing your hand on any part of Dennis' arm was like touching the steel cables used to hold up a suspension bridge.

My kids would always look forward to visits from Uncle Dennis. Back then he would make appearances on the Letterman show and Regis & Kathie Lee. While in our area he would also perform in schools, churches and gymnasiums.

One display of strength that would always astound me was with a 100 pound dumbbell. With his arm braced against an incline bench so he couldn't swing the weight up, I would hand him the 100 lb bell. He would execute 10 perfect curls. To this day I have never seen that done by any human of any size. Inconceivable!

And in '92 I became Dennis' 1st student. I was putting together a show to present to kids in schools and strength feats were an excellent way to get attention. At 39 I was a bit skeptical about how much strength I could add since conventional wisdom then said that after your mid-30's rapid strength decline is inevitable.

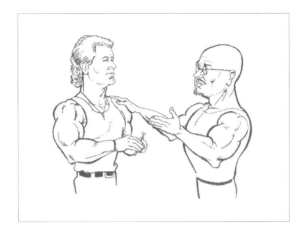

But Dennis trained me from my elbows down to my finger tips as well as between my ears. After a couple of years I was bending steel, tearing decks of cards behind my back, rolling up frying pans and holding tremendous weights. Freaky Forearms became my descriptive.

From Harvard Health- A strong or weak hand grip carries more than just social cues. It may also help measure an individual's risk for having a heart attack or stroke, or dying from cardiovascular disease.

As part of the international Prospective Urban and Rural Epidemiological (PURE) study, researchers measured grip strength in nearly 140,000 adults in 17 countries and followed their health for an average of four years. Each 11-pound decrease in grip strength over the course of the study was linked to a 16% higher risk of dying from any cause, a 17%

higher risk of dying from heart disease, a 9% higher risk of stroke, and a 7% higher risk of heart attack.

The connections between grip strength and death or cardiovascular disease remained strong even after the researchers adjusted for other things that can contribute to heart disease or death, such as age, smoking, exercise, and other factors.

Interestingly, grip strength was a better predictor of death or cardiovascular disease than blood pressure.

Is grip strength a measure of biological age?

The findings from the PURE study aren't new. Previous research has also linked grip strength with future disability, death, and the onset of cardiovascular disease in adults. But this is the largest study to have made the connection. The fact that grip strength was a relevant measure across high-income, middle-income, and low-income countries lends credence to the findings.

An individual's age in years (chronological age) can be quite different from his or her biological age. Although there's no exact definition for biological age, it generally indicates whether the body is functioning better or worse than its chronological age.

Many things influence biological age. Key factors include overall physical fitness, the presence or absence of certain medical conditions, and muscle strength.

The PURE study suggests that simply measuring one's hand grip strength could be a good way to assess biological age- "grip strength might act as a biomarker of ageing across the life course."

The researchers suggest that weaker muscle strength makes it more likely that a person will die sooner if he or she develops a chronic medical problem, compared with those who have more muscle strength. In other words, muscle strength could be good for survival.

From Reuters- Strong grip may predict longer life at all ages

(Reuters Health) - Grip strength may be a better predictor of future health than some measurements doctors currently use to gauge risk, a large UK study suggests.

Although grip strength has long been a good indicator of frailty or health in older people, it could help doctors understand adults' risk profile at all ages, including the odds of heart and lung disease, cancer and overall mortality, the study team writes in the British Medical Journal.

"Grip strength is easy to measure and may be useful in helping to predict future disease," said senior study author Stuart Gray of the University of Glasgow.

"Grip strength showed a stronger association with cardiovascular disease than blood pressure and physical activity, which was a bit of a surprise," Gray told Reuters Health by email. "It highlights nicely just how strong the association is."

The researchers studied more than half a million participants in the UK Biobank project, who were aged 40 to 69 years when they were recruited in 2007-2010. Periodically over the years, participants underwent medical exams, provided samples and answered extensive questionnaires about health and lifestyles.

Gray's team also tracked participants through medical records for an average of seven years. During that time, more than 13,000, or nearly 3 percent, had died, while close to 6 percent developed heart disease, about 2 percent developed respiratory disease and close to 6 percent were diagnosed with cancer.

After accounting for age and a wide range of other factors, such as diet, sedentary time and socioeconomic status, the researchers found that muscle weakness, defined as a grip-strength measurement of less than 26 kilograms (57 pounds) for men and less than 16 kg (35 lb) for women, was associated with higher overall risk of death and higher risk for specific illnesses.

Each 5-kg (11-lb) increment of grip strength below these thresholds was tied to a 20 percent increase for women and a 16 percent increase for men in the risk of death from all causes.

For death from heart disease, the risk increased 19 percent for women and 22 percent for men. For death from respiratory disease, the increase was 31 percent for women and 24 percent for men, and for deaths from all cancers, the increase was 17 percent for women and 10 percent for men.

Overall, the researchers note, people with the lowest grip strengths tended to have lower socioeconomic status and were more likely to smoke, to be obese and to have higher waist circumference and body fat percentage. They also ate fewer fruits and vegetables, exercised less and watched TV more.

Skeletal muscle's critical role is often underrated, the researchers write. It controls body movements, serves as the body's primary protein store and plays an important role in regulating blood sugar.

"This isn't just about frail adults . . . This is important for adults in the prime of their life," said Carrie Karvonen-Gutierrez of the University of Michigan School of Public Health.

"If this is a robust indicator of underlying disease risk, we should consider incorporating it into clinical care . . . particularly in areas around the world where we have limited resources," she said.

Researchers have also found that grip strength can be a good overall marker for aging. In Norway, for instance, researchers found that elders' grip strength in their 80s and 90s can predict the likelihood of making it into the 100s.

From KRON4- Why Grip Strength Predicts Your Longevity

If you're like most people, you don't think about your grip strength until you struggle to open a jar or untighten a knob. But now there's reason to know your actual grip strength.

What a Strong (or Weak) Grip Says About You:

Research shows your grip strength is a good predictor of overall strength; and overall strength is a good predictor of overall health.

According to a four-year global study of over 140,000 people aged 35-70 years old in 17 countries, a weak grip is a stronger predictor for death from ANY cause compared to systolic* blood pressure. In other words, a firm, strong hand grip is a better health assessment tool than your blood pressure.

These findings were published in The Lancet, a peer-reviewed medical journal, and were broadly consistent across various countries and economic levels.

How to Measure Grip Strength:

Muscle strength is measured by grip. Your handshake can reveal your health status. Do you have a weak handshake or are you known for having a "vice grip"?

Grip strength testing is inexpensive, easily performed in a doctor's office, and the results are immediate. NOTE: Grip strength is affected by a person's stature:

⇒ Circumference of the forearm

⇒ Circumference of the hand

⇒ Hand length

Since stature affects grip strength, relative grip strength is a better method of assessing muscle weakness (i.e., comparing changes in strength) vs. absolute grip strength using standard normative values.

Powerful Predictor of Death:

The researchers found that every 11-pound decline in grip strength was linked to the following:

16% increase in death overall

17% increase in both cardiovascular and non-cardiovascular death

7% increase in the risk of myocardial infarction

9% increase in the risk of stroke

Grip strength may be a biomarker of aging where the loss of grip strength might be a good marker for underlying age-related disease.

Frailty and Survival:

Grip strength is useful for identifying frailty among patients. In the aging population, frail status based on grip strength is associated with:

⇒ Comorbidity (when two chronic diseases or conditions are simultaneously present in a patient)

⇒ Cardiac risk

⇒ Sarcopenia (age-related muscle loss)

Low muscle strength predisposes individuals to fatal outcomes when chronic medical problems occur, such as cancer, type 2 diabetes falls, fractures, & respiratory illnesses. Although grip strength was not associated with developing these conditions, muscle strength could be good for survival.

From Readers Digest- Strong hands, strong heart? Does grip strength show life expectancy?

Your heart is about the size of your fist. Recent media reports suggest that as well as telling you something about the size of your heart, your hand can tell you your stroke, heart attack and death risk.

What has grip got to do with life expectancy?

This idea is not new. After the atomic bombing of Hiroshima in 1945, studies were carried out on thousands of survivors, testing all aspects of bodily function over many years. Radiation did not affect grip strength; however, a surprise finding was that grip strength in general was a strong indicator of life expectancy. In a separate study starting in 1965, involving thousands of World War 2 war veterans living in Hawaii, grip strength again seemed to go hand-in-hand with life expectancy.

The largest study to date, involving nearly 140,000 people in 17 countries, reported in 2015 that people with lower grip strength had a higher mortality rate and were more likely to suffer a heart attack or stroke. Grip strength was even suggested to be a more accurate test than blood pressure! And you have to hand it to the researchers: they did not include those who became ill soon after the study started in their results. In this way they could be sure that poor grip strength was not simply the consequence of a pre-existing condition which shortened the participant's lifespan — we all know how weak we become as soon as we are ill.

Anyone for grip training?

Grip training is gaining popularity, and real contests take place called 'World's Strongest Hands' and 'Mighty Mitts'. Events include ripping phonebooks in half and bending metal horseshoes into hearts. A word of caution, however: strong hands do not always indicate a strong heart. Especially not in the case of some bodybuilders who have used anabolic steroids for strength and died tragically young of a heart attack.

From Science Daily- Hand grip strength may be associated with cardiac function and structure.

Better hand grip strength may be associated with cardiac functions and structures that help reduce the risk of cardiovascular incidents, according to a study published March 14, 2018 in the open-access journal PLOS ONE by Sebastian Beyer and Steffen Petersen from the Queen Mary University of London, UK, and colleagues.

Hand grip strength, often used as a measure for muscular strength, has been previously associated with risk for cardiovascular incidents and mortality. However, little is known about the association between hand grip strength and the shape and function of the heart.

Beyer and colleagues gathered and analyzed cardiovascular magnetic resonance images and data on hand grip strength from 5,065 participants that were previously participants in the UK Biobank prospective cohort study. They then constructed a statistical model that accounted for potential factors that could impact the data such as baseline demographics, cardiac risk factors, drivers of muscle mass, and physical activity level.

The researchers found that participants with stronger hand grips were often pumping more blood per heart beat despite having a lower heart mass, indicating that the heart is suffering less from a condition called remodeling (reshaping) of the heart muscle (remodeling can occur in response to stressors such as high blood pressure or a heart attack). Less remodeling is known to reduce the risk for cardiovascular events. The authors suggest that these findings help improve our understanding of how heart shape and function may contribute to the association between handgrip strength and cardiovascular emergencies and mortality.

"Our study of over 4,600 people shows that better handgrip strength is associated with having a healthier heart structure and function," says Petersen. "Handgrip strength is an inexpensive, reproducible and easy to implement measure, and could become an important method for identifying those at a high risk of heart disease and preventing major life-changing events, such as heart attacks."

So what I have gleaned from the research as well as my personal experience is that a smart arm and grip workout is way more beneficial to overall health than the nonsense we are being sold daily. Conventional Wisdom has everyone fretting about getting in their 'cardio' work. What a joke. Especially the way 'cardio' is implemented with motorized machines set to raise ones heart rate up to a 'target zone'. Or sad joggers plodding along the roads of America in search of the 'runners high' and a lean physique while only really getting a beat up body from all the pounding on the uneven concrete.

I'm not saying not to work your entire body. Actually no matter what body part I may be focusing on, ALL my exercises are full body exercises. And because of this I get a full cardiovascular effect from everything I do. And that includes Grip Training.

Pinch grip training, crushing grip training, and holding grip training create overall hand strength. Dennis Rogers had me train all 3 ways.

For example I would be pinching 2 Olympic plates smooth side out for time. Or pinching an old style York dumbbell end and either holding for time or tossing it up in the air and catching it with the other hand. Years ago in some of my live presentations I would set 2 different sized dumbbell ends on a bench. I called them Blobs and the challenge was to have someone from the audience come up to lift the Blob straight up and grab the money under it. One weight was about 25 pounds and the other 35. You wouldn't believe how many guys couldn't even lift the smaller one. And I'm talking about guys with big gym muscles who could bench press a lot of weight. The guys who did hard manual work were able to lift them and get the money. If grip strength is such a predictor of good health into the future, why are the vast majority of gyms across the country not addressing it? Why aren't Physical Education classes teaching and encouraging kids to 'get a grip'?

For crushing work I would use a set of Captains of Crush grippers or an IronMind adjustable gripper. And either do varied sets and reps or just hold them closed for time. Even simple things like grabbing a full size newspaper sheet and rolling it in my hand until it was a tiny ball were very effective.

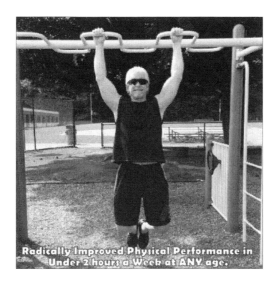

Radically Improved Physical Performance in Under 2 hours a Week at ANY age.

Holding myself up on a chinning bar or with parallel handles for time is a great warm up for your body as well as fantastic grip work. Lifting and holding a loaded barbell or heavy dumbbells is great as is a farmer's walk with anything heavy--

those big water jugs they use for the office coolers are fun to take a walk with.

Then to support the hands Dennis had me doing wrist work as well. And the way I have my home-made wrist roller set up I can get my heart rate elevated very quickly while developing my grip as well as forearms. Palms up dumbbell wrist curls with arms resting on your legs is awesome for forearms as well.

Other than our face, our arms are the most displayed body part (hopefully :D). A smiling, friendly countenance leaves a great impression while a well-defined arm on either a man or a woman sends a powerful message. You really can't fake what the condition of your arms is saying. Makeup, a tan and injections can temporarily pretty up a face but your upper limbs are either there... or not. And now with all the research results, we know that at the end of those well conditioned appendages are grips that dramatically improve our overall health.

While the grip work improved my function, the bicep has always intrigued me. As a youngster back in the 1950's my Grandpa would always ask me to 'make a muscle'. I would lamely hold up my little arm and squeeze. He would laugh and tell me how strong I was getting. And now that I have Grandchildren I do the same thing.

Of course there is way more to strength and fitness and health than an old bicep. But when flexed it is a thing of beauty. And a gnarly tricep muscle is required as a sort of platform for the bicep. Above will be a well rounded deltoid and below a sinewy, hard wire, sometimes freaky forearm.

Being lifetime Anabolic Steroid and Performance Enhancing Drug free, growing a set of 'guns' took some hard, consistent, and smart work. Gaining size and strength in the upper arm is not just a matter of pumping up or going for the burn. As with the rest of training it all starts with position. Have you ever noticed guys or girls who curl a ton of weight yet have neither size or shape to their biceps? Bad position is usually the main culprit.

And for function you would want an arm that does not detract from overall performance be it in a sport or in life. High load, high volume and high velocity are important factors in training. My training not only increases the size of the muscle (hypertrophy) but also promotes new muscle cell growth (hyperplasia). Even from a vanity standpoint this is good news. Your arms will look fantastic all the time, not for just the 1 hour after you leave the gym!

My favorite upper arm movements are:

Standing Straight Bar Curls, EZ Curl Bar Curls, Alternate & Simultaneous Zottman Curls, Preacher Curl Iso Holds, Wall Ropes Bodyweight Curls and Holds, Dips on Vince Gironda Dipping Bars, Supine Tricep Extensions (Skull Crushers), Towel Tricep Pulldowns, Wall Ropes Standing Tricep Extensions and Statue of Liberties.

And the ways to execute the exercises are:

Extreme Slows, Rebounds, Altitudes, Iso's, Quick Stops, Isometrics, Explosive Power, and Max Strength.

With so many ways to develop and maintain grip strength, I try not to be conformed to training in a particular place or using particular equipment or even at a particular time. During the long drives across Pennsylvania and beyond on my way to see my youngest son wrestle in college, I developed a Driving Workout. (Please note that I am a very experienced driver and stayed totally focused on the road and my surroundings.) While all the positions, holds, and movements involved my entire body, my hands got some serious work. I would arrive at my son's match totally pumped up! However, I better check with my older son who is in law enforcement and maybe a lawyer before teaching this workout! :D

And finally you can make it all fun as well. With some consistent work bending big nails in half, tearing decks of playing cards and old phonebooks, rolling up frying pans into a tube and twisting horseshoes into heart shapes will all be within your ability. Now when reading that, if your 1st thoughts included 'that's impossible!' or 'I could never do that!' then you are just like I was.

And THAT is why I really needed a teacher and mentor like Dennis Rogers. He actually lives the old Napoleon Hill principle, 'Whatever the mind can Conceive and Believe, it can Achieve.' Once my head got right, the training was easy.

Intelligent Strength is the answer in Exercise. Be in Position and Train Hard. Everything else is just minutiae. We can all rationalize just about anything and that is so true in how we exercise. The conversation in our heads leads most down the wrong road. *We cannot 'negotiate' our health.* Worrying about the scale or the mirror or anything else just distracts us from the task at hand. Our bodies will adjust our muscle and fat levels accordingly. All the while reflecting our new-found level of fitness.

The man who taught my son and me so much about training actually proved it dramatically. The beauty of his system is its simplicity. Phenomenal results are attained in minutes a day and not hours. Instead of being mindless while exercising or taking ridiculous rest periods between half-hearted strength sets, this system of exercise just wants your total focus for a short period. Some people balk at that but it's the only way to make progress toward your goals.

During training Jay Schroeder teaches about actually how to focus. He uses the acronym PIPES. Exercise needs to be Physical, Intellectual, Psychological, Emotional and even Spiritual. Please don't let total focus scare you. It will actually help you to more deeply relax and even sleep better.

Just like most of us have a difficult time admitting when we are wrong, so does our culture. It's science finally admitting that the whole egg is really good for you. We have to admit that the way we exercise & what we think we know about exercise has been wrong or at the very least- extremely inefficient.

Just for a minute can you imagine mastering a small number of exercises? And then imagine that those exercises done regularly will allow you to enjoy every aspect of your life more fully? You will be strong, healthy, at your best bodyweight and look good in a swimsuit. And you will not spend hours a day but minutes a day to reach this place. I allowed myself to buy in to this system and forced myself to unlearn so many exercise programs & philosophies that could not deliver in the long run.

Get in Position & get after it! Reject Mindless Exercise.

Going back to the caveman, did our ancestors have to slowly warm up and stretch out when the week's food supply was passing by? Or did he see the beast, grab his spear and go all out so he could feed his family? Our ancestors were ready for anything. It was a mindset. When our minds are right, we are always ready for action, be it physical or mental. No warm ups required.

YOU MUST CREATE AN EXTENSIVE DISTURBANCE OF HOMEOSTASIS IN ORDER TO ELICIT A HIGHER LEVEL OF SUPERCOMPENSATION.

TRAIN with EMOTION (Game/Match Level) & with a Picture of the RESULTS YOU DESIRE.

The exercises are called Isos and are executed with a continuous 'pulling into position' for the entire time.

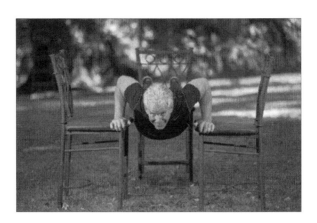

The 4 main benefits of this type of training are:

1. One's Range of Motion increases proportionally with strength thus preventing injuries.

2. Hyperplasia occurs in that more cells are recruited which causes an increase in muscle density. Conventional training would cause more muscle size (hypertrophy).

3. Contractions that take place to hold you in position are at high velocity- the same as if you were moving at maximum velocity.

4. Muscles are fed energetically the same as if you were out running at max speed.

If you stop & think for a minute; this is quite amazing. How fast can even the top runners in the world go all out 100%? Maybe 20 seconds & they have to start pacing themselves.

What condition would you be in if you trained yourself to be able to go at Max Velocity for a full 5 minutes? And ANYONE can do it if they so desire.

Athletes of all ages should pause and think about this. *Get stronger and skill improves regardless. Don't train skill without having a base upon which to grow, as strength is the limiting factor in every movement.* When your foundation improves, everything above it becomes more solid. And if you're going to sign up for private lessons, make sure you can balance on one leg, squat, bend, rotate, and push/pull all while breathing through your nose, or else you're better off throwing your money into a fireplace- at least you'll be able to start a fire.

It's tough to find a starting point sometimes. The way we are doing these particular movements really shows where our weaknesses are -- even for super trained professional athletes... egos come into play because everyone wants to feel good working where they are strong... but strengthening the weak links is best in the long run... -RJ

We have to be careful in designing exercise programs that the movements go towards strengthening the bodies' weak links and are not just difficult for the sake of being difficult. -RJ

In 1972 a Philadelphia Eagles football coach told Jay Schroeder- 'What should I do in the weight room? Never go in a weight room unless what you're training for is to be good in the weight room. Go out and get yourself a real job- a farmer, a brick layer- that's where you're going to develop your muscles in Harmony with each other and it will make you a better athlete. In a weight room you get too specialized and develop more injuries.'

OUR BODIES WERE CREATED TO BE ABLE TO MOVE IN A BALANCED, STRONG AND GRACEFUL WAY... THEREFORE, WE ARE ALL ATHLETES IN THE GAME OF LIFE...

THE GREATEST SINGLE PREDICTOR OF A PERSON'S HEALTH AND LONGEVITY OTHER THAN GENETICS IS HOW MUCH PHYSICAL WORK THEY DO.

Training should be preparation for the future. What I see is activity only in the moment and most of the time that activity is more than worthless even harmful to the present as well as the future. -RJ

Generally speaking, most exercise equipment like treadmills & ellipticals as well as other gym machines are bad for your neurology as well as for your full musculoskeletal development.

Minimal Exercise with Maximal Focus yields the Greatest Benefit! This 'truth' hit me yesterday after 40 years of 'working out' in all different types of training systems & philosophies.

I'm really trying to get somewhere! #EarthDay

While a great workout at the gym can be exhilarating, there IS something about doing 'other than your normal' activities that can take you to another dimension.

Chopping wood the old fashioned way brings one to a place of solitude as well as awareness of things often ignored... It's not a 'mindless' pursuit, it does bring all types of stimulation to the senses--- the visual splash of wood chips, the sounds outside oneself of the birds & breeze, the sounds within of increased respiration & heart function, the feelings in one's hands, arms & torso... AND then the payoff... the timing of which cannot always be predicted...

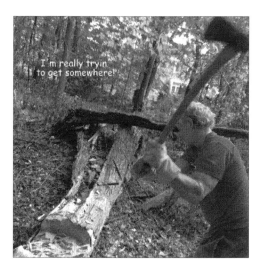

Leaning on the axe, wiping sweat, feeling the quiet returning to one's innards & considering all of Nature's might that went into growing the tree. But wait! All the effort it took to chop through just 1 part of 1 tree & I can see thousands more.

Every time a huge tree falls out in the forest behind my house, it seems that a handful more sprout up in the same area. A Great Gardener is looking after those trees. ☺

Gym question--

If I carry large bags of peat moss,

holding on with only my fingertips--

Must I still 'hit the gym'????

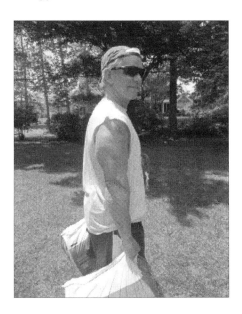

Rolling in the Hay... or Rolling Hay! ☺ At least 10 years ago, my now Gorilla youngest son & I rolling a 1,000 pound Hay Roll that was rotting & soaked with rainwater.

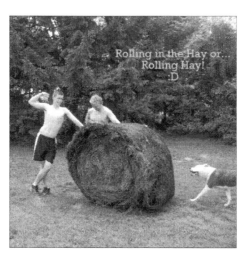

Yikes! If you want to get your heart pumping & your delts burning-- the next time you're driving through some farmland & see a huge hay roll-put on the 4ways, jump out, run into the field & push it as far as you can then wave to the Farmer thanking him for the best 30 seconds of heart-exploding-in-your-chest feeling you have ever had! ☺

The now-legendary Paffenberger findings should give you a huge clue when trying to figure out the FITness puzzle. What is the greatest predictor of a person's health-factors and longevity other than genetics?

What you eat or when you eat it?

How much water you drink?

How much sleep you get?

Your percentage of bodyfat?

How far or fast you can walk, jog or run?

How athletic you are?

How stress-free your life is?

How many cardio or aerobic or stretch or yoga or tai chi or pilates classes you take a week?

White bread/whole wheat, chemical sprayed/organic, caff/de-caff, red wine/lite beer, sun/shade?

The answer to all the above is a resounding No. <u>THE GREATEST SINGLE PREDICTOR OF A PERSON'S HEALTH AND LONGEVITY OTHER THAN GENETICS IS HOW MUCH PHYSICAL WORK THEY DO</u>. In other words, how many calories you burn directly affects your present and long-term health. The optimal workload per week is from 2,500 to 3,000 calories.

Health & Wellness- Old School Fitness

Pick a Card--- ANY Card!

The major component to fantastic health for you and your family is exercise… and we all know that as a culture we do not get enough of it. We can sit back and blame technology in all of its forms but the truth is WE are responsible for our family's fitness.

Back in the day it was about being outdoors for hours on end in all seasons physically DOING stuff. We really did WALK to school… and back. Shoveling snow was expected as was cutting lawns (with a push mower!) along with all kinds of chores. But that was then.

It amazes how parents bring their young athletes to me and that 13 year-olds cannot execute 1 perfect push up. Think about that. But ask the child and they will tell you they can do 20 or 50!

My son was the same way. The coach would command everyone to get down and 'gimme' 10 pushups. Maybe 1 kid would have it almost correct… the rest looked like a bunch of sway back cows dipping their hips in unison. And poor position ALWAYS limits athletic performance and makes us more susceptible to injury.

So what can a Parent do? It should be obvious that the Crawl, Walk, Run model should ALWAYS be used when exercising. Master the correct position 1st then move on to more complex tasks.

I will teach you 2 movements that will aid your child to become stronger and more athletic...and greatly reduce the chance of injury.

Here is an idea that has been used in various ways through the years. Use a deck of playing cards. # cards are worth their face value, face cards are worth 15, Aces 20 and Jokers 25.

Clubs & Spades are for a lower body exercise- the Wall Squat. Hearts & Diamonds are for the upper body- the Push Up. If you do not take the time to learn how to Perfectly execute these movements- do not proceed since you will not be helping your child.

Wall Squat- feet hip width apart, toes forward, distance from wall is determined by sliding down to thighs parallel to floor- knees should be slightly over top of foot, execute by pulling self down with hamstrings, head-upper back-low back stay in contact with wall, chest is spread with traps & hands relaxed, bottom position is below parallel just before low back pulls away from wall (YES that deep!), keep pressure on entire foot into floor to keep hamstrings activated at bottom, be sure to keep pressure with the adductors so knees keep in line with feet/hips, hold for appropriate time.

Push Up- feet hip width apart, hands a tad wider than shoulders, imagine a bar under both hands to keep them straight, imagine pulling the bar into the bottom of your chest (solar plexus) to keep position, traps down, elbows at 45 degrees from body, up on feet with torso flat, execute by slightly bending elbows and imagine pulling the floor to your chest- no movement other than contracting the Lats & Biceps hard while also contracting the Glutes (buttisimo in Italian :D), hold for appropriate time.

Shuffle the deck. Take a card. 3 of Hearts? Push Up position, contract appropriate muscles hard- 1 Mississippi, 2 Mississippi, 3 Mississippi.

Take a card. Ace of Spades? Perfect Wall Squat at bottom, all muscles activated- then 20 Pink Elephants.

As a family during TV commercials- 1 hour show gets 17 minutes of exercise. During School work- set the timer, 3-5 minutes of exercise every 15 minutes…

Once you lose position, the exercise is over. Work up to an entire deck at once. Incredible strength will be gained by the entire family.

4

SLEEP

Sleep Fitness

As some chase the promises of the Fountain of Youth, the rest of us would settle for longer, active middle years before we get really old. Billion dollar industries have emerged to keep us 'Forever Young' but seem doomed to ultimate failure.

Therefore, to dramatically extend the active middle years, we will have to lead a somewhat disciplined life. *Eating smart, training smarter, sleeping smartest and doing whatever it takes to keep a positive, hope-filled attitude does not seem too big a price to pay for those who aspire to live a long, happy, productive life.*

Personally, it seems I was always burning the candle at both ends. Part of it started as a form of rebellion during my youth after being forced to go to bed at certain times. My Mom's wisdom regarding 'getting a good night's rest' was ignored in favor of late-night must-see TV and endless social commitments that always materialized 'After Midnight'.

My college years were worse but I easily transitioned into the bar ownership years when Sunrise meant go to bed. Then the 'not ever missing an opportunity to watch or play with or do anything at anytime for my Kids' years almost killed me.

Sleep was so erratic but I never gave it a second thought because I thought (wrongly) that I could make up for it by eating right and training regularly and taking mountains of nutritional supplements. It didn't work.

Real sleep deprivation appears to be one of the biggest culprits in our fast-paced, high-tech modern life. Sleep is not 'wasted' time. We are designed to need restorative time that allows our body to stay functioning at optimal levels.

The release of certain hormones like Seratonin (the feel-good hormone) and HGH (Human Growth Hormone) are two of the main benefits of restorative sleep. Sleep supports neurological performance, endocrine balance, immune system functioning, and musculoskeletal growth & repair.

It appears that we humans are wired to get the highest quality sleep when it's dark and that optimal sleep time for adults is 7-8 hours.

The 2 ways that we can dramatically improve our sleep are by upgrading our Sleep Environment and Behavioral Conditioning.

The Sleep Environment is upgraded by having the best mattress and pillow you can afford, deluxe sheets, a cool room temperature, the room as dark as possible, no snoring mates, no pets in bed, no leaky faucets, etc. In other words, stop at nothing to make your sleep environment as sleep-friendly as possible.

Behavioral Conditioning is about learning some new habits and developing rituals to transition into a deep, restful sleep. While some believe in taking pharmaceuticals to sleep, I prefer a more natural approach since I don't like a drugged feeling. Herbal teas, melatonin, or 5-HTP (5-Hydroxytryptophan) would be options for re-setting your sleep clock.

Do a bit of research on these 2 things… and even insomniacs will benefit greatly.

Sleep is an incredibly active time for our bodies and brains when we undergo all manner of growth and repair processes through a dynamic biochemical orchestration. When we know the facts on sleep, we're more likely to give it our full respect.

A full night of sleep will enhance your memory performance and creative problem solving skills the next day, not to mention make you a better person to be around by helping you see the positive in your interactions. Additionally, a good night's sleep will further boost your athletic performance, including speed, accuracy, mood, and overall energy.

And you might be surprised to see those extra pounds you just can't seem to shed... vanish.

If you don't sleep enough, the cortisol levels rise in your body, which makes it really easy to gain that unwanted belly fat. But when you sleep for many hours at a time your body produces human growth hormone (HGH), which helps you to lose fat and gain muscle. Also, when you don't sleep enough, your ghrelin levels are increased, which means that your body just wants to eat. This is the hormone that kicks in to let you know that you're hungry. When you don't sleep, your body overproduces this, so you tend to end up eating more than you should.

In addition to that, the hormone leptin gets suppressed when you don't sleep enough. This is the hormone that tells your body you've had enough to eat.

Taking drugs to get quality, restorative sleep is never the answer!

This is what is working great for me.

⇒ Tone down all electronics & artificial light for 1-2 hours before sleep time.

⇒ Brew a cup of Trader Joe's well rested herbal tea or sleepytime, let steep for 5 minutes.

⇒ I either eat with or throw into the tea 3 squares of Trader Joe's 72% Belgium dark chocolate.

⇒ I also eat ¼ cup serving of plain gelatin that I prepared or just throw it in the tea (1/2 tsp).

⇒ And take my bed time gut health supplement-bentonite clay.

⇒ & finally I rub Magnesium oil into my ribcage. (Taurine works great as well- 1- 500mg tab 30 mins before bed).

⇒ Get in bed and Read something positive & uplifting---Sweet Dreams!!

5

FOOD -KEEP IT SIMPLE-

After Christmas one year it was decided to get another dog since Grace our German Shepherd was getting old. We have had many dogs over the years, some mutts & some purebreds, most were rescues.

Somehow I had stumbled on a breed called the American Bull Dog. I read some amazing stories about the dogs and started to look around online. I found a 10 month old dog in New Jersey and we went to check him out.

It was Mom and Dad along with our 2 youngest, Krissy and Buddy. And we brought Grace since we would need her approval (or at least reluctant consent) to bring another pet into the home.

Well we always had what we thought were big dogs but this was a Big Dog. He looked like a Pit Bull on steroids but with what seemed to be a very Good Attitude. As most rescues, he had a sad history but we were willing to take the chance.

Naming him on the way home was great fun. We settled on the name Rev which is short for Revelation which was in a current hit song that came on the radio.

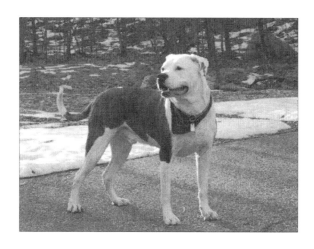

So Rev grew over the next few months to about 125 pounds! He looked very muscular. He got along with Grace who finally passed and he got along really well with our cat, Jazz.

I remember taking him to one of those big pet stores up by the mall to get some supplies. Everyone wanted to meet Rev! Especially girls & women. Goodness gracious I had a line of females follow me out to the parking lot, ages 8-88. He was the consummate 'chick magnet'.

A guy from church named Brother Derrick had loved American Bull Dogs since he was born and he strongly encouraged me to get this special dog food for Rev. The only place he knew to get this special food was a place in Newark, New Jersey called Ace Pet which is at least a 45 minute drive for me.

Well I get there and it's in a part of the city that you wouldn't want to go to at night. Literally it was on the 'other side of the tracks'.

So Rev and I walk in. The place was like an old warehouse with low ceilings and very cool pet stuff everywhere. But the place looked nothing like the fancy pet store up by the mall.

Brother Derrick had given me the names of the 2 owners. But before I opened my mouth, the guy standing behind the raised counter looked down at Rev and said 'that's a pretty old dog'.

I politely replied that Rev was only 5. The counter guy looked down again and said 'he's fat!' I felt my pressure begin to rise. Who is this guy calling my dog fat? It's like calling my mother or wife or one of my kids fat... even if it's true maybe you could gently suggest the idea?

After I took a breath, I met Jesse- one of the owners. He pointed to a picture on the wall of an American Bull Dog in full extension on a jump. He said that if they don't stay narrow through the waist, it will lead to hip problems when they get older. Although Rev was strong enough to carry the extra weight, it just wasn't healthy.

So I purchased the special dog food and left with a plan from Jesse on how to get Rev's weight down to where it should be.

My boy wasn't too happy about the food restriction. In fact at one point, he snuck in a neighbors garage and ate an almost full 20 pound bag of cat food!

But we stayed the course and within 6 weeks Rev went from 124 pounds down to 104. A 20 pound weight loss! He looked fantastic!!

So I read the label on the dog food a bit closer. I knew it was all natural but never really looked close at the ingredients. Totally grain free, no GMOs, nothing artificial. Depending on which formula you get the 1st ingredient is either real meat, fish or fowl. Lots of vegetables. Some fruit. Lots of good fats.

Hmmm. Since I have been a student of Health, Fitness, & Wellness for just about my entire life, I had been considering going to an eating plan called Primal. It is exactly like the dog food formula Rev was eating.

So I started to eat that way. No, not dog food. And after about 6 weeks, guess what? I had lost 20 pounds as well!

And Rev and me lived happily ever after. Just something to consider...

Eat smart

Don't be a victim of processed foods or familial eating habits. The foods you eat can either add to your health & sense of well being or take away from it. A body that has to work overtime to digest is a stressed out body. Eat to nourish, repair and energize. Don't let old habits ruin your health and add to life's regular problems. If you think you know how to eat but are in terrible shape or have to be on medications then 'you really don't have a clue'.

Humble yourself. It's okay to need help. Seek out someone who exudes health & wellness not some 'expert' who does not look like they are taking their own advice. An older person would be a better choice here since the cumulative effect of what they believe will be visible. Be open to wisdom in this area.

Processed Foods means food that has been cooked, dehydrated, frozen, dried or smoked. Many nutrients like vitamins and enzymes are usually destroyed this way. Junk foods are actually *designed* to make us want to eat more of them-- large processed food companies actually have "food scientists" who study addiction and *intentionally* engineer their foods to appeal to those natural human cravings. One is never satiated eating these 'foods'.

80

Food Sensitivities or Allergies are usually pretty easy to determine. The usual culprits are gluten, grains (rice, quinoa, buckwheat, barley, oats, corn), legumes (beans, and especially soy), some nuts and seeds, dairy (pasteurized milk, cheese, yogurt), and eggs. Many times I've found that a compromised immune system can make us sensitive to foods or it might also be a faulty digestive tract. I would go strict primal with your eating for a month or so & then try adding foods back in.

Or just eliminate the suspect foods for 21 days and see how you feel. It's usually a grain like wheat or pasteurized cow's milk or sugar in its many forms. I remember when I eliminated wheat—no more bloating or sleepiness after meals…

Also note that Caffeine stimulates your cortisol production and adrenaline and makes your liver push out glucose. Basically it makes your blood sugar rise in the same fashion that sugar would. So since I like coffee I usually drink it with a healthy fat like organic cream or organic coconut oil or organic unsalted butter. Drinking it this way, the big blood sugar rise is avoided.

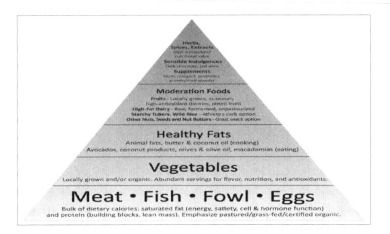

Look closely at this food pyramid and you will discover some reasons you aren't losing weight or feeling great. Consuming **fat does not make you fat!**

To determine where you are with your eating right now it might be wise to use a daily food log program to see what type and how many calories you are consuming. But you will only have to count them for a short season. When you are physically working hard and you know which foods to eat, how much you eat will eventually just fall into place. For example when I shovel snow for 4 hours my body will crave more food that day. The next day I might not be so active and I will naturally eat a bit less.

Vegetable and seed oils became dietary staples in the '60s and '70s when animal and saturated fat started getting a bad rap. We now know that animal and saturated fat are critical components of a healthy diet, while industrial seed oils pose the riskiest threat.

Hydrogenated or partially hydrogenated oils — including soy/soybean oil and canola oil — are made up of highly processed unhealthful polyunsaturated fats that can lead to a number of health problems, including higher risk of heart disease and diabetes, hormonal disruption, immune system damage, increased risk of allergies and asthma, and interference with healthy fat metabolism. Likewise, vegetable and seed oils go through extraction methods that render them unnatural and full of inflammatory properties that wreak havoc on health.

So what oils are safe for consumption and cooking? The best oils for cooking are:

Coconut oil, Palm/palm (kernel) oil, Butter/ghee (from grass-fed sources), Beef tallow, Pork lard, & Duck fat.

Healthful dressing oils include: Olive oil, Avocado oil, & Macadamia oil.

Keep It Simple!!!

I remember when one of my daughter's was getting ready to go into 9th grade. She needed a doctor's physical in order to compete in sports. We went to our Pediatrician with the necessary forms.

When it came time to pay the bill, the Doctor's office charged us an extra $50. I called the next day and was told that since they had not seen our daughter in 8 years, her records had been put in storage. And the extra $50 was to dig out the old records!

All of our children were blessed to have very healthy childhoods. Some might call it luck or good genetics. I believe it came down to food and drink choices my wife and I made for them & large amounts of physical activity.

My wife always said that if we could get high quality food in them 80% of the time everything would work out.

The problem for parents is defining Quality Food and Drinks. You'll have a good idea if your family is eating 'right' by how they look. 81% (get used to that number ☺) of what you look like is based on what you eat. The other 19% comes from genetic makeup and activity level.

A Family Meeting is in order before making any major changes in how you will eat (I can see my kids rolling their eyes 'Another Family Meeting, Dad?' LOL). Parents need to decide the direction of their families and if the family is off track, it's time for a change. Explain all of the benefits of eating healthy and commit to it yourself.

At the risk of inciting passions about the type of diet one should follow — Primal/Paleo, Vegan, Low Fat, Fast Food, etc., I'll give you some general 'food philosophy' that should be basic to all. This reiterates what is on the food pyramid.

The majority of my calories come from pastured, grass-fed, organic meat, fish, fowl and eggs. Protein is the building block for the body including developing lean mass. The saturated fat provides energy, satiety and impacts cell & hormone function.

Locally grown and/or organic vegetables provide optimal nutrition and antioxidants.

Healthy fats should come from avocados, olives, extra virgin olive oil and macadamia nuts. We use organic animal fats, butter and coconut oil for cooking.

Locally grown fruits in moderation can be a great source of antioxidants especially berries and pitted fruits. My 'go to' fruit is the apple.

Nuts, seeds and nut butters are great snack options. Young athletes can add starchy tubers and wild rice for additional quality calories.

Another moderation food would be fermented dairy such as yogurt.

What are called Sensible Indulgences would include dark chocolate and red wine.

If you want to find out which foods might cause you trouble, just eliminate them for 21 days and see how you feel. It's usually a grain like wheat or pasteurized cow's milk or sugar in its many forms. I remember when I eliminated wheat — no more bloating or sleepiness after meals...

Sometimes moving toward optimal health can be a bit inconvenient in the beginning. But once the family 'buys in' to the idea it's easy to find fresh and economical food sources. Aside from our own garden, we try to buy vegetables and fruits locally in season. Local farmers' markets abound.

Our chicken and eggs come from a local farm where we buy in bulk for ourselves and about 20 friends. Farmer Tom out in Hackettstown, NJ raises all natural beef and 'we go in on a cow' with friends.

Since New Jersey has too many lawyers and thus so many laws, we cannot get raw milk which is an awesome food. So every time I drive out to Pennsylvania I buy raw milk on a state inspected farm. Then I follow in the steps of the great bootleggers during Prohibition and bring raw milk, yogurt, cheeses and ice cream back to Jersey. My Great-Grandmother actually did run 'bathtub gin' from Hoboken, New Jersey up to Nyack, New York with the stuff under her floorboards during the time of Prohibition! I don't have floorboards so I just bring it over state lines in coolers in the back of my SUV.

Be creative with your meals. With the profound impact food has on our very existence, consider making food selection and preparation a centerpiece of daily activity in lieu of 'time wasters' that try to convince us of their importance on our lives (ie- technology essentials, 'must see' TV, etc.)

The goal is always 100% 'on track' eating BUT if one 'falls off the wagon' just get back on as soon as you can.

Ohhh-besity

Back in 1973 I had dropped out of college for the 1st time and I was working full time for a large company in my hometown of Secaucus, NJ. Although I had been a star athlete in high school, I had never 'worked out' before. Noticing my rapidly declining health and overall poor physical condition, it was apparent that I had to do 'something'.

Well the guys I worked with would tell me stories about a local legend who had gone on to become Mr. America and Mr. Universe. The stories inspired me. One of the men loaned me 2 dumbbells and I would go home after my 3-11 shift, sit in front of the TV watching Johnny Carson and move those 'bells anyway I could think of until I was exhausted. As my body changed for the better so did my attitude and the rest is history.

I was fortunate enough to meet the source of my inspiration this past year- 33 years later. His name is Dave Draper- the Blonde Bomber. Before Schwarzenegger, Draper was on the cover of all the muscle mags and in the movies.

Dave sent me a letter recently and I just love his writing style. This Particular Message is timely for all of us. I really think it could be a huge hip-hop or rap hit!

Draper here... Hello, Obesity. Sit. Have a Donut.

They are told, but nobody listens. The word is out, but they do not respond. It's in the news, but none heed the message. Magazines inform, newspapers report, the television declares and the internet details hard-hitting facts, embarrassing truths and alarming consequences, but the points are ignored.

Obesity kills. Eat right. Exercise regularly. Be responsible. Teach your children. Be aware: Diabetes, heart failure and cancer lurk...

...Have we descended too far? Have we gone downward too long? Is the momentum too great? Is there no turning back? Have we lost our will, our way? Are we weak and numb, ignorant and lazy?

The overweight exposé has grown long hair and fangs and howls like a wolf in the town square. Rather than correct a wrong or prevent a disease, cure an illness or aright a social aberration, we have ignored it, we have apologized for it and perpetuated it. Obesity, weight-impairment, is linked to -- the result of -- caused by our misdirected childhood, the stresses of living, global warming, pesticides, environmental anomalies, the unconscionable fast-food industry and carbon footprints in the sand.

Please, spare me the pathetic details. You ever see the size of the sit-read-compute researchers making these obscene postulations? They're humongous, I betcha. They love their French fries and Big Gulps.

Moreover, we (they, rather; hunky pc society, hungry business opportunists, overweight-activists, governmental grant researchers) have arranged alternatives and conveniences to accommodate what is largely a weakness (lack of control, absence of discipline, need for distraction, apathy), leading to an epidemic of costly diseases (heart problems, diabetes, cancer) which shorten lives, discourage or trump preemptive resolutions and raise insurance rates and medical costs across the board.

The problem: We eat too much, we eat the wrong foods, and we don't exercise.

Solution: Exercise, eat right, be responsible.

I sound like I'm high 'n mighty and I'm ranting 'n raving. Not! Well, maybe just a little. I'm mostly a concerned observer with his own dysfunctions who sees a landscape of neat kids approaching their teens on the brink of disaster. They're happy, innocent rolly pollies about to face the consequences of their up-to-now acceptable (normal, I'm sorry to say) condition. Before long, buds, it's show time.

I see young guys and gals struggling with their excess weight. It's obvious in their cumbersome movements, their timid self-consciousness, their feeble efforts to keep up, their adopted or contrived bullyness, or their painful shyness. I see it in their eyes, especially the confused and desperate eyes of chubby young girls, and it breaks my heart.

Shame on us. Fatness is a mistake, not an accident, and we've led them to its commission... we propagate the troubling condition.

Guys can handle it. Overweight can be disguised as big. They can use it on the football field. They can wear XL pullovers that say Broncos on the back. They can lean on lighter kids. Girls can't. Guys have lotsa testosterone. Girls don't. Guys are guys. Girls aren't. Thank heaven.

Girls are responsible for more important things like bosoms and bottoms and small waists. Their girlfriends admire such attributes, society acclaims them and dopey guys drool over them. I, of course, am simply an innocent bystander.

... We are partners all, striving and applying, falling and rising, trying and failing, living and learning and growing and succeeding.

We're okay. I'm talking about those adults outside our cosmic gym, who are not tuning in, the kids beyond our invisible fitness bubble unaware of their physical trouble. The number of heads cannot be counted and is increasing day by day.

It makes me mad and sad. The problem is a big problem, collectively and individually, because it's been a work in progress for a long, long time. The stomachs protrude like beach balls, and they are neither fun nor funny. They didn't appear overnight. They're major construction projects, serious developments.

I'm sounding like a mean guy (a bum, yes -- mean, no), but the problem is larger than oversized midsections.

Where's the basic human intelligence, the common sense?

Where are the personal responsibility, healthy pride and self-control?

Where are the minds, hearts and souls?

Where are the parents and role models, schools and educators?

Where's concern for self and the whole, one's people, one's nation?

'Draper here... Hello, Obesity. Sit. Have a Donut'

Daydreamers beware. A concerned overweight person ought not to seek to be slick, svelte and sassy. Not yet, later maybe. He or she ought to take wise and comfortable steps to lose weight and condition him or herself regularly, day by day, every day, for good. Remember and never forget: The rewards are instant and constant and reap dividends forever. Seed-sized efforts for a vast harvest of achievement. Think big where it counts.

Again, the causes of common obesity are simple: poor food choices, poor eating habits, over-consumption and inactivity. Certain… of us …might attribute their oversized problem to proper eating habits gone north and vigorous exercise gone south. Discipline, alas, is not their foremost quality and devotion to the cause of leanness has been known to disappear like chocolates.

Here's all you need to know, my concerned overweight friends:

It's got to do with exercise and eating right and wrapping your arms around yourself with affection. It includes encouragement, endurance and common sense; faith, hope and love. You possess them all or you wouldn't be here, wherever that might be. Dare I say it, no self-loathing and negative imagery, ever. Neat trick, good luck.

The eating thing is no secret -- more balance and less indulging. Eat less of most things and stop eating the wrong things; more living foods and less processed foods, more muscle building proteins and fewer fat-building empty carbs, and no greasy fats, ya rats. Eat smaller balanced meals more frequently, increase water consumption and add a quality vitamin-mineral supplement daily. No booze, no smokes, no soda pop, no whining.

Neither is the exercise thing a covert operation -- more vigorous activity and less idleness. … it works, as does a dripping faucet in filling buckets. The faucet is adjustable, by the way.

Life, besides being unfair, is full of inconveniences. Eating right and blasting it can be dern near impossible in the world of opportunity -- overtime, kid's soccer practice, finals, holidays and the beer and ice cream in the fridge.

We need tools, aids and armaments to succeed. Will, desire, need and certainty are the handy tools in our toolbox for effective construction. Self-control, persistence, compromise and smart planning are the feathered arrows in our quiver if we're to hit the target, the bull's-eye.

Ah, but there's always a tempered glitch. The causes of jiggles and tight jeans can sometimes be complicated: hormonal, metabolic, glandular and genetic. Here excuses are not necessary. We have reasons.

Whoever, whatever, whenever or why, the stubborn predicament must be attended. The overweight condition has a way of becoming a permanent condition the longer it accompanies us and grows comfortable.

If I was 30 to 70 years old and about to mount the bucking bull -- roller coaster if you prefer -- of weight loss, muscle building and conditioning for the first time since the launching of the Ark, this is what I'd do:

1. Reality check -- I'd recognize the seriousness of the matter, make a commitment to resolve it and set a realistic goal. I'd prepare for compromise and hard, loving work regularly.

2. I'd exercise every day for 30 to 60 minutes (what a relief!)...

3. I'd dig up some basic nutritional info... and outline a high-protein, medium good fat and good carb, low-cal diet and follow it like a puppy follows its best friend -- eagerly, innocently, lovingly, always and everywhere. You know this stuff, just do it!

4. A routine can be... simple...That's all. Work up to it over time. Enjoy the time, drink of its incalculable worth and remember: It's more important than most everything else you do. It supports and adds years of quality to every facet and fiber of your life. Don't hurry your workout, don't chase it away, enjoy it. It's here and now. It works.

5. Let your light shine.

Feels like spring in Central Cal. Good weather for plucking daisies and doing tailspins. Don't try these activities at the same time... without practice, goggles, a nose guard and collision insurance... a fistful of four-leaf clovers, one rabbit's foot, a lucky penny... feeding the pets, saying goodbye, canceling travel plans, confessing your sins...

Go... Look up... Dave

Emotions- get to the bottom of your emotional reasons for eating^^^

6

WATER

When we have athletes who are working very hard the suggestion is 1/2 your bodyweight in ounces = Daily Suggested Water Intake.

But should it be based on Thirst?

Drink smarter-

Keep it pure. No sugar, no artificial sweeteners or flavorings or colorings should be added. Be aware of how one becomes dehydrated. Dehydration makes the body feel stiff, de-energized and sluggish. Add some fresh fruit or pink salt or your own minerals to clean water so that it's absorbed into your cells more effectively. It's easy to stay hydrated.

My personal pet peeve- folks who walk around with a huge jug of water.

Drink when you are thirsty. Too much water flushes out valuable minerals.

We all know the saying 'an apple a day keeps the doctor away'. Actually an apple a day (or 2 of if you drink dehydrating beverages) is a much more efficient and healthful way to stay hydrated.

Apples are over 80% water. The water in fruits and vegetables is way more effective for cellular hydration than plain water. For most people all the extra water does is make them pee more often while doing next to nothing for true hydration.

If you are eating foods loaded with garbage and drinking beverages loaded with garbage, dehydration is a real possibility. However, rarely will one become dehydrated doing some work or training hard.

Think about it before you buy into the stay hydrated-drink sports drinks with electrolytes- sales pitch. Or drink a gallon of water a day scam.

There has never been a time in history when massive amounts of water had to be consumed while incredibly hard physical work under extreme conditions got done. So now the question is whether science has showed us a better, healthier way to live by consuming liquids even before we thirst... or are we all getting hosed by slick marketing that seems to make sense?

I drink about 3 cups of organic coffee with some sort of fat in it just about every day. Caffeine can dry me out a bit and I'll notice that I get thirsty. So then I will drink some water as described or eat an apple. Many times I find that more than dehydrating me, too much coffee will cause a need for more Vitamin B complex. So I'll just pop a sub-lingual tablet under my tongue and I'm good to go.

When athletes come in to heal fast from injury, I suggest 1/2 their bodyweight in ounces as the Daily Suggested Water Intake. And they are training super hard during a time when their bodies are trying heal as well. Most folks I know or see train never come close to this type of hard work.

If your performance is off, there are so many other factors to consider before you need to 'hydrate more'.

Opening a can of Seltzer>>> the hard way!

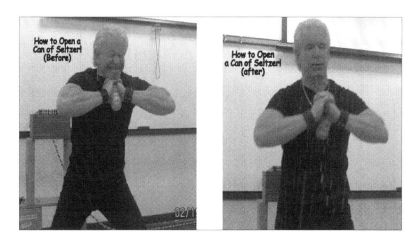

Don't drink soda boys & girls... it'll weaken your bones-- among other things. ☹

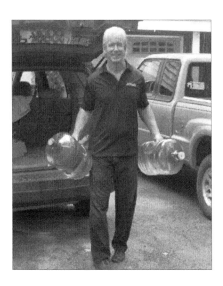

Ready to hydrate? I think it's a very personal thing. Some folks go around chugging gallons a day.

I hate a ton of water sloshing around inside. Even though some disagree, I think thirst is a great indicator of how much h2o we need.

Either way, carrying the jugs as pictured is great. As an exercise it's called a Farmer's Carry. Just schlep a heavy thing in each hand until your grip fails, rest a bit & repeat. Great Workout!

MICRONUTRIENTS & SUPPLEMENTS

I have been through many supplement regimens over the years-- sometimes relying only on food by itself, other times mega-dosing with vitamins, & other times only on herbs.

It appears that our bodies are under almost constant attack from a variety of sources. And while we have a phenomenal capacity to ward off diseases of all sorts, I believe that whenever possible we should take positive steps to bolster our immune system. In addition, detoxifying from contaminants we are regularly exposed to is also a good idea. The level of contaminants in the air we breathe, the water we drink, the food we eat and on and on is dizzying.

My present philosophy is to gird up all my body's systems & not get caught up in the 'latest, greatest' supplement game to treat specific maladies.

We must all remember that the benefits of organic eating & natural supplementing usually take 'time' for the desired changes to take place.

The 'cumulative' effects of a wise lifestyle will occur if we can patiently wait. In our 'instant gratification' world where pharmaceuticals are looked to for a 'quick fix', it can be our biggest challenge to wait for the 'good seeds' we are planting in our bodies to take root & then bear 'good fruit' —robust health!

Here is what I presently take- full explanations as to 'why' would fill a book but, suffice to say, that this is all really good stuff.

While eating as Clean as possible what is today referred to as a Primal/Paleo diet, this is the list of extra things I take:

Minerals are critical and the only place plants can get minerals is from the soil. If the soil is depleted, you can get lots of vitamins but very little minerals from your fruits and veggies. I take either liquid minerals or my friend Stephen Santangelo has some great home-harvested minerals as well. I use Stephen's on my morning eggs in lieu of salt...

Baking Soda w/o aluminum helps to keep your body's PH in a good place. I take 5 grams a day.

Organic Apple Cider Vinegar is a digestive aid & is high in potassium. I take 2-3 tablespoons a day.

Organic Tumeric is well-known for its anti-inflammatory, antioxidant, anti-microbial, anti-malarial, anti-tumor, anti-proliferative, anti-protozoal and anti-aging properties. I take

1/2 tablespoon up to 1 tablespoon a day with a bit of black pepper for better utilization.

Coconut oil is amazing. Here are some of the reasons: Proven Alzheimer's Disease Natural Treatment, Prevents Heart Disease and High Blood Pressure, Treats UTI and Kidney Infection and Protects the Liver, Reduces Inflammation and Arthritis, Cancer Prevention and Treatment, Immune System Boost (Antibacterial, Antifungal and Antiviral), Improves Memory and Brain Function, Improves Energy and Endurance, Improves Digestion and Reduces Stomach Ulcers and Ulcerative Colitis, Reduces Symptoms of Gallbladder Disease and Pancreatitis, Improves Skin Issues (Burns, Eczema, Dandruff, Dermatitis and Psoriasis), Prevents Gum Disease and Tooth Decay, Prevents Osteoporosis, Improves Type II Diabetes, for Weight loss, for Building Muscle and Losing Body Fat, for Hair Care, for Candida and Yeast Infections, for Anti-Aging, and for Hormone Balance.

I use it for cooking, oil pulling teeth and gums, as an after shave, on my hair and in one of my cups of daily coffee.

Men starting around 45 or so will naturally have a drop in testosterone levels. In order to slow the process down I alternate between *Organic Maca* powder and *Fenugreek* every few weeks.

One of my good friends knows the Longevity Sage, Peter Ragnar. His daily herbal mix is *He Shou Wu* 1/2 tsp, *Epimedium Powder* 1/2 tsp, & *Tongkat Ali* 1/32 tsp.

Whey Protein is my protein powder of choice for times when I'm just not getting enough from my diet. I use an unflavored product that can be added to just about anything that mixes easily. Those with severe milk allergies might try an egg protein.

Vitamin D3 I only take during the time of the year when I cannot get 20+ minutes a day of sunshine. 10,000 IU per day during the winter seems about right. Look for D3 serum to ensure supplementing with D gets down to the cellular level.

Nordic Naturals Omega-3 is the best. I take a daily teaspoon especially during the winter months.

Vitamin B is only taken on an 'as needed' basis during high stress, not enough sleep, high caffeine, rundown times. The one I prefer is a sublingual B complex.

Salt is not a supplement per se. But *Himalayan Pink Salt* is actually good for you…. & it can be used for periodic internal cleansings.

Creatine monohydrate is something I should mention in case you catch me with it someday. As I've gotten older (65), I've noticed that my muscles do not seem to hold water as they did in my youth. I've been taking creatine for about 10 years in small amounts (5 gm/day) and notice zero performance improvement but for vanity purposes, it does the trick.

If you have had to take anti-biotics or have undergone chemotherapy or radiation, it might be a good idea to use a few gut health products for a season. I prefer fermented foods, kefir, yogurt and clay.

Bentonite Clay is an age-old method of treating many different disorders in a number of cultures. From the skin to the digestive system, this substance has the ability to fight infection, boost immunity and more.

If you choose to consume bentonite clay, be sure to do it only in small quantities and use clay sold by trusted merchants. I use the Living Clay brand.

A friend, who is sometimes referred to as the Witch Doctor by the athletes he treats, has me mix 2 ounces of clay with 16 ounces of water in a container you can seal & shake vigorously. After mixing you open the container to let the clay breath for at least 10 minutes. I take 2 ounces 1st thing in the morning and right before bed as well. So every batch lasts me 4 days.

As I was being encouraged to write this book, I noticed a pain in my right hip flexor. Over the next week it got worse to the point that it was waking me up in the middle of the night. I tried everything I could think of to no avail.

Then one morning after a shower I noticed swelling in my lower abdomen just above where the pain in the hip flexor was. Yikes! I saw a client then went to an Urgent Care facility.

The intake nurse was taking my vitals and marveling at the great shape I'm in for 65 years old. I'm smiling at her & thinking 'If I was in such great shape, I wouldn't be here!'. The physician comes in and examines me. She declares that it's probably an inguinal hernia. I told her I hadn't been lifting anything that had caused any tearing sensations. She wrote an order for an ultrasound test to confirm her findings.

I raced to get the test done since I was a bit concerned. I've never had a hernia before & I still do Strongman feats. A lovely lady with a heavy Russian accent performed the ultrasound. Because of the location of my discomfort & how thorough she had to be, normally private things were no longer private. What else can you do but make a few jokes & bear with it?

When she announced 'I can't find anything' (add accent), I totally cracked up. Of course she had meant she couldn't find any sign of a hernia. By the next day the Urgent Care place had the report. They then ordered a cat scan with contrast which I had the next day after drinking some really nasty looking stuff.

I read the report late that afternoon and it has words like possible colonic mass, diverticulosis, liver hemangioma, and enhancing lesion. What???

Since part of my 65th birthday celebrations had involved getting a complete physical exam, I already had an appointment with a Gastroenterologist the next week. He looked at the reports and scheduled a colonoscopy for a few days later.

Now colonoscopy jokes are always funny until they might be looking for something serious-- in you! I at least tried to lighten up the somber mood of the waiting room but no one who is fasting & thinking about the test is ever really in a joking mood.

Anyway all the Doc found was a benign polyp. Even so, I wasn't too happy to have any polyps. I knew that something was missing all along. Gut health is vital. The probiotics and digestive enzymes I took were not getting the job done.

I went directly to a friend who is affectionately known as the Witch Doctor. He has been dabbling in all sorts of natural products that one might use for all sorts of maladies. He has been telling me to take clay for years... but I never got around to it.

I've always tried to get what I need nutritionally from the food I eat and then only supplement as needed. So I'm usually wary of adding another pill to my diet unless absolutely necessary.

But gut health is so vital for so much and what I was doing was inadequate. The Witch Doctor gave me some clay, told me how to mix it and how to use it. It has worked wonders in helping to completely digest food as it detoxifies my entire body.

And I slept well that night. And the hip flexor pain was gone! No hernia. I searched the literature on polyps and could not find any connection between my gut issue and hip flexor pain. Go figure.

Gelatin is very good for you. Good old Knox is fine. If you're doing bone broth and chewing on the end of organic chicken bones on a regular basis, you won't need gelatin. I take ¼ cup serving of plain gelatin that I prepared or just throw 1/2 teaspoon in a beverage.

Serrapeptase is a proteolytic enzyme. Called the Miracle Enzyme it's been around for a number of years and it comes with a myriad of benefits:

⇒ Helps Treat Pain and Inflammation

⇒ Lowers Risk for Atherosclerosis

⇒ Kills Bacteria and Promotes Wound Healing

⇒ Treats Respiratory Infections

⇒ Fights Autoimmune Diseases

⇒ May Help Treat Neurological Disorders (Including Alzheimer's)

⇒ Treats Bones and Joint Pain/Infections

I take it on an empty stomach for all or any of the above conditions. I've also taken it with food to aid digestion for those times when I overeat or over-indulge on the Jones Family comfort food of choice- Ice Cream!! Research it yourself. It really is amazing.

Following this regimen of supplementation for 12 months should resolve any allergies or asthma or other seasonal illness, at least in my experience.

A Day in the Life EXAMPLE:

Upon arising: a 2 oz serving of Bentonite Clay, followed by a glass of pure water (with fresh lemon or lime juice & a smidgen of organic stevia is optional), followed about 30 minutes later by a cup of organic coffee with 2 Tbsps organic grass-fed butter, cinnamon and ginger. An alternative to the butter is organic Coconut Oil or organic 1/2 &1/2.

Depending on my schedule and how I'm feeling I might then have a serving of fresh organic fruit with my Special Drink- ½ tsp Baking soda, ½ tbsp Tumeric with black pepper, 3 tbsp Apple Cider Vinegar, 5g creatine, 10-20 grams of whey protein, man herbs from above list, and 1tsp of maple syrup. I would also add 1/4 tsp liquid minerals if I'm not taking mineral crystals on my food. Use pure water to make the drink but be careful when adding the baking soda, ACV and tumeric- things can get explosive!

Sometime later: 3 whole fresh eggs cooked in organic coconut oil, organic bacon fat or organic butter with green salsa & hot sauce to taste along with Himalayan salt, pepper and a pinch of Santangelo's Minerals.

Take 1 tsp Omega-3 oil & 1,000IU Vitamin D3 serum (not needed during summer months if you are getting plenty of sunshine).

Rest of Day/Night—plenty of organic protein, organic veggies & good fats, water when thirsty.

Serrapeptase on an empty stomach or full depending on my needs.

Follow 81/19 rule—get it right at least 81% of the time & don't beat yourself up about the rest.

Sleep- This is what is working great for me. Tone down all electronics & artificial light for 1-2 hours before sleep time.

Brew a cup of Trader Joe's *well rested herbal tea* or *sleepytime*, let steep for 5 minutes.

I either eat with or throw into the tea 3 squares of Trader Joe's 72% Belgium *dark chocolate*.

I also eat ¼ cup serving of plain gelatin that I prepared or just throw it in the tea (1/2 tsp). straight from the packet.

And take my bed time gut health supplement- clay.

& finally I rub *Magnesium oil* into my ribcage. (*Taurine* works great as well- 1- 500mg tab 30 mins before bed).

Get in bed and Read something positive & uplifting--- Sweet Dreams!!

Rundown or at the first sign of oncoming illness you have a choice- all 4 are very effective--

Wellness Formula by Source Naturals (I prefer the capsules if I can find them) or *Airborne* or *Sinu Oregano* in the nose & *hydrogen peroxide* in the ears...

Brother Brian Smith's Good-for-What-Ails-Ya Elixir:

2 ingredients- *Organic Ginger-* 2 palm-size pieces & *Organic Garlic-* 2 bulbs

Wash & cut up Ginger into teaspoon size pieces (approximate).

Get as many Cloves out of the Garlic as possible.

Put both into a pot with 2 quarts of fresh H2O.

Cover, bring to a Slow Boil and let simmer for 15 minutes.

Ladle out a cupful while hot, *Organic Honey* to taste, sip slowly while deeply inhaling steam.

Re-heat & repeat every few hours until symptoms subside.

Brian says you can re-use the ingredients a few times until you can taste it weakening.

We store the extra liquid and ingredients in a Mason jar in the refrigerator for future use.

I got excellent results clearing up a deep sinus infection…

Also great for Colds & Flu & as a general Detoxifier

Also please remember that supplements are meant to supplement a fresh, organic whole food way of eating and drinking!

8

INJURIES & ILLNESSES

Overcoming Injury At Any Age

Before beginning or continuing any exercise program it is critical to understand the role that injury plays in you being able to achieve your fitness goals.

One of the realities of life is that from time to time we all suffer an injury. And if it's not too traumatic we can actually finish the game or whatever physical thing we are doing. However, injuries not properly dealt with lead to us developing 'compensation' patterns that put us at greater risk of further trouble.

For example when I was playing sports as a teenager I had many ankle sprains. Ice them to get the swelling down, tape them up tight and get back in the game or practice… right? That's what I did but I found out years later that the improperly healed ligaments in my ankle were leading to a myriad of other problems- knees, back, hamstrings, etc.

I kept 'compensating' for all of my injuries in a variety of ways until physical activity was not fun anymore.

But this is what I learned a few years back. What controls your structure is your muscles and what controls your muscles is your nervous system. So it's critical to see how your nervous system is controlling your muscles.

I use a technique to see if muscles are firing properly. I go around your body and test different muscles but I'm not testing to see how strong you are. I want to see if your muscles are able to turn on and turn off at the right time. This will show us how well your nervous system is controlling that muscle.

That's important because the way that your muscles support your body and protect all of your joints is by Absorbing Force. So whenever you do an activity- sit in a chair, brush your teeth, walk, run- force is going to be entering your body and your muscles are going to have to be able to turn on in order to absorb that force.

Now if your nervous system is slightly imbalanced or has some kind of abnormal reflex and it's not able to turn on the muscles at the right time, that muscle is not going to be able to absorb that force and that force is going to travel to another area--- like a tendon or a ligament or a disc in your neck or back or cartilage or meniscus or labrum or bursa, fascia, bone or some other muscle. Most structures are not designed to Absorb Force.

When force is transmitted to an area where it's not supposed to be, it going to cause damage to that tissue. And that's when you're going to start getting sore or developing scar tissue or inflammation or stretching and fraying, degeneration of a disc or a bulge or herniation. You'll start to develop problems that all stem from the same thing- your body not able to Absorb Force properly.

This is very important to understand because even the simplest movements can be very painful for many of us. Even the doctor's prescription to 'walk more, it's good for your health' can be a very tough assignment. *We all need to learn that 'mind-less' activity is not the solution to long term health.*

So if I test all of your muscles and I find 1 or 2 or maybe even 5 muscles that aren't turning on properly, then I have to figure out which part of your nervous system is not doing what it's supposed to. Once we figure that out then we can actually do therapy or treatment that can stimulate that part of your nervous system and get it to start working again. Once it starts working it's going to turn on all those muscles and those muscles are going to start absorbing the force so that it doesn't go into your neck or low back or wherever you're hurting.

At that point those areas can actually start healing. Right now any time you do any kind of a therapy or strengthening activity all force is going to transmit into the injured area and cause it to be irritated. And that's partly why your pain is not going away. So we're going to get you to be able to absorb force properly and then we'll take you to the next step to get the injured tissue to heal very quickly.

We have a therapy called the ARP, which is an electrical modality which runs a current through you that is harmonious to your body. So if we would put the direct current on an area where there was no injury, the current would just flow right through you and you'd just feel a light tingle. (please note: this is not electric stim or tens)

But we take the pads and start searching around on your skin and when we get to a place of disrupted tissue or scar tissue or inflammation, the current can't flow through that area and you start feeling it a lot more. So that gives us a tool where we can actually search around and find where that damaged tissue is. That's very beneficial because a lot of times someone will feel pain in one place but when we put the pads on that spot they hardly feel anything. But then we move the pads around and a person can actually feel where the source of the problem is.

So what we do then is start running the current through the area and have you go through some movements. The current is designed to break up scar tissue. Whenever you have an injury, your body is going to bring inflammation into that area and scar tissue is literally going to wall off that injured tissue. If you have a wall of scar tissue around that injury, you can't get blood to flow through the area. AND without blood flow, you're not going to heal very quickly.

So what the ARP does is break down that scar tissue and floods the area with blood and healing occurs very quickly then. Typically it takes about 4 sessions to get the inflammation out so you don't feel it like you did the first day.

THEN we need to build up the strength that you've lost in the area. Whenever you injure an area, you're going to compensate with other muscles and so you'll lose a tremendous amount of strength around the injured site. And getting the area stronger will help prevent re-injury and when trained properly, your muscles will be able to absorb a tremendous amount of force.

Dr.'s Office

Consider this during the flu season and the rest of the year as well.

A friend of mine is a doctor and I had occasion to pick something up at his office. While waiting, I noticed a 1-page paper lying by the magazines. The premise of the article was that we often hold on to 'false beliefs' which are detrimental to us.

The writer observed that our society firmly believes in an 'outside in' approach to sickness and health. We're taught that something 'out there' makes us sick- a virus, bacteria, pollutant, stress. When this 'something from outside us' makes us sick, we need to turn to another 'something outside ourselves' to make us well- a drug, surgery, remedy, etc. This belief places our power outside of ourselves and makes us 'victims' of disease dependent upon the intervention of something external in order to be 'well'.

Continuing the author states that Health and Healing are really 'inside out' jobs. Louis Pasteur, the father of germ theory, stated toward the end of his life 'It's the soil, not the seed that matters'. *This means that it's the state of your body, not the germ that determines whether you'll be sick or healthy. Germs and bacteria do not cause disease.*

A sick weak body is susceptible to pathogens (bacteria and viruses associated with illness), just like rats congregate at the garbage dump because the garbage is already there. If it's clean, there's nothing for them to eat and you won't see them.

The writer goes on to state that even with degenerative and autoimmune disorders, it's the state of the body which will determine the state of our health more than anything else. It makes much more sense to spend our time and energy doing all that we can to increase the state of our health and trust the healing power within our body than to hope we can dump solutions into the problem once it occurs.

I don't know how a simple stop at the doctor's to pick something up could turn into something so deep and thought-provoking. Of course the writer over-simplified his point of view BUT somewhere in there is the simple message that we all need to exercise regularly, eat the most natural food possible, take a few supplements for insurance and keep a positive outlook on life.

And please don't ask me 'But did you get your FLU shot?'. I wouldn't want to stir up any controversy with my answer- LOL. Fight for YOUR Health!

From one of my friends to you-- We do know that inflammation, especially chronic, systemic inflammation seems to be involved in nearly every disease under the sun. Obesity, cancer, heart disease, autoimmune disease – if it's killing people, increasing health care costs, and reducing quality of life, inflammation is bound to be involved at some level. That makes things easier, in my opinion, because we have a good idea how to avoid chronic inflammation, and that should take care of half the battle.

Crippling Back Pain does not have to stop you!

Back in the 1980s when I was in the bar business I started getting neck pain that really got my attention. As you can imagine, having 'live' entertainment 4 nights a week, not closing until 3am, after hours shenanigans, and going to bed when the sun came up was not the healthiest of lifestyles. But at 27 years old the body can withstand a lot... until it starts to break down.

It started with not being able to turn my head. I visited a local chiropractor who took an x-ray and showed me how one of my cervical vertebrae was at least 50% displaced. From my history in sports he said it could have come from a hit in football, which sounded possible. (As the years have gone by, I always wonder if he showed everyone the same x-ray!)

So the chiro manipulated my neck for a few visits and then gave me something that EVERY chiro should do. He gave me specific exercises. I did them religiously and the problem resolved itself.

Then a few short years later I developed pain in my chest. I had changed occupations by then and was training people. One of my clients was a doctor who specialized in internal medicine. She determined that the agita and heartburn and general pain was as a result of a hiatal hernia! I had to look up what it was.

After a few dietary modifications, I was fine in no time.

Then a year after that I started getting really severe low back pain. During one of these episodes that would last a week or more I was hurting so bad I couldn't get off the floor. Eventually an MRI showed a few disc herniations. I tried a chiropractor, physical therapy, massage, heat, ice, stretching, injections and wearing a corset. Nothing worked and the bouts seemed to be getting more frequent & more intense.

A friend had just had back surgery & was encouraging me to go that route. And it looked really bad. Here I was supporting my family as a fitness trainer & I was a physical mess. To drive to see my clients I would first put on a binder under my clothes to hold my back tight. Then I had a big dark blue reusable ice pack I would put over the binder and hold that in place with a lifting belt!

I would arrive, put on my happy face and ask if I could leave my icepack in my client's freezer while we worked out. During those years I had about 19 clients who I drove to see multiple times a week.

In my head I had decided to go the surgery route. One of the women I was training was an accountant and a weekend warrior tennis player. She made me promise to get and read a book by a doctor she had gone to in New York City.

Later that morning I staggered into a Barnes & Noble Bookstore and bought the book. I had a meeting about an hour's drive away so I strapped on my icepack and took off. The temptation to find out the 'secret' in that book was too much to bear so I started skimming through it... while driving on the New Jersey Turnpike!! (at least I wasn't texting... um that wasn't invented yet- whatever).

By the time I reached my destination, I had found out enough to really think what was being proposed might actually work. In the parking lot I shed my lifting belt, icepack and even my binder (corset). I was a bit tentative walking into the meeting but I survived and then drove home like a normal person without props. And 2 days later I was squatting with 300 pounds on my back and it felt great!

I would call what happened 'miraculous' but it wasn't really a miracle. It was me discovering more about how my body functions than I knew before. The answer to my pain was not in a pill or an injection or surgery or stretching or how herniated my discs were.

Think about this. First of all, there was no blunt force trauma to my back- no bones were broken. Secondly, injuries heal yet mine kept coming back which really makes no sense. If you cut yourself and start to bleed, what do you do? Put pressure on it until the bleeding stops or get a few stitches. Then you might cover it with a bandage and it will start to scab over. Then it might turn colors as it continues to heal. Finally the scab will fall off and you might have a scar.

That's how things normally heal. But what about my back? The pain coming and going over the course of weeks and months is not normal. So what was triggering this abnormal response? I believe the old neck problem, the hiatal hernia and my low back pain all came from the same place.

A daily battle for me has always been fear, anxiety, worry, discouragement and how to deal with the stress that life brings. But over the years I've learned ways to combat all this stuff. And I'm able to wake each morn with a new hope for the day and the future. But mental and emotional things absolutely affect our physical bodies. And the big way we know this is by experiencing pain, from mild to excruciating.

And left unattended this pain will begin to have tremendous influence on our lives! You can imagine how just moving your body is affected. Pain can alter your thought-life! And your emotions change in how they respond to just normal life situations or conversations. So it's a really big deal for the vast majority of people I know and meet... if we're all being honest.

So how was my neck, chest and back pain related? The pain was all in what I would call classic locations for pain from stress to manifest. For many stress can allow the body to be overcome with a myriad of diseases, but for me it was structural pain.

The doctor's observations and my symptoms and the ultra-sounds and X-rays and MRIs all saw a herniation or inflammation. *But the source was never diagnosed. What needed to be fixed was not where they wanted to cut.*

My reaction to the stresses of life was the problem. But that is so hard for us to admit, never mind believe. Because it means on some level we're a 'head case'. We want a drug or a surgical procedure to fix us. But many times the surgery just opens up the door to other painful areas. Then what? Your movement patterns have changed so now your entire body is out of balance. You compensate so the wrong muscles are working to get you from point A to point B.

And I was anticipating pain. As soon as I felt a familiar little shock in my back, I would automatically lock up by holding my breath and getting really tense. And the cycle would continue. And I would never get better.

I had a huge turning point event in 1992. I had heard a speech years before where the speaker said 'faith and fear cannot live in the same body at the same time'. What the...? It took me a week to figure out what it meant. Something will control your life, faith and belief or... fear!

Now it's quite easy to hear that and say it sounds good. It's entirely different when you have to physically respond. It's either called 'faith and belief in action' or 'that's really scary, let's get the heck outta here!'

There is no compromise either. You must be 100% all-in. So that night back in '92 had me for the 1st time in my life go that 100% all-in. It changed the course of my life... and my back pain.

With regard to my back, it amounted to gaining knowledge and then overcoming fear. For example, did you know there was a very large back pain study in Europe years ago using x-rays and MRIs? They found that for all the people who reported moderate to severe back pain with disc degeneration and herniations, there was an equal amount with the exact same diagnostic reports who had no symptoms at all. How could that be?

Sometimes a diagnosis can cripple you. My back pain would come and go. The most severe injuries bring pain that never lets up. I came to understand what triggered my pain. I addressed it and do so just about every day of my life. I move about freely. I lift heavy things. I do not wear a brace or a special belt. I'm not on drugs & do not run to a chiro, physical therapist, masseuse or acupuncturist.

In this vast world with so much information available, I believe we must be able to shut out the noise around us and be brave enough to look inside ourselves.

Dr. Caroline Leaf, the great cognitive scientist puts it this way. 'Our thought lives have incredible power over our mental, emotional, and even physical well-being. Our thoughts can either limit us to what we can believe we can do or release us to experience abilities well beyond our expectations. When we choose a mindset that extends our abilities rather than placing limits on ourselves, we will experience greater intellectual satisfaction, emotional control, and physical health. The only question is... how?'

So much of what is in this book brings us to that answer. The Grandmaster Strongman of this generation Dennis Rogers has helped me find and release strength I would have never believed I possessed. Jay Schroeder's training system pulls all our humanity together in a world that keeps moving toward being mind-less.

How I eat and supplement supports the physical body which supports our minds and emotions. *It's really quite simple but it is also unarguably cumulative.* It's an everyday thing.

129

We can figure out the source of your injuries and put you in the optimal neurological and musculo-skeletal position and get you strong. And the correct innervation of your entire body will help your body even combat illness.

Learn how to get in the proper positions and keep moving... every day.

Direct Current Speeds Healing! Do NOT mess with AC current in water!!!

DC Healthy☺ , AC Deadly ☹

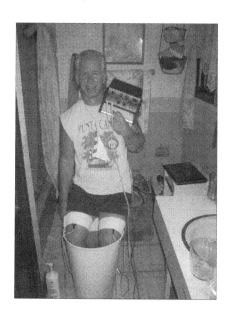

1980- 6 months after Major Surgeries on 3 Limbs.

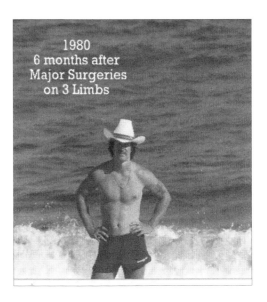

Motorcycle crash! Shattered left elbow & severed left tricep, ACL & MCL left knee, 12" x 6" hole in right shin, All ligaments torn in right ankle-- ☹

Hospital for 30 days. Did my own PT because I had to.

Doctor's quote- 'If you had not been in great shape BEFORE this accident you probably would have died or at least never been able to return to normal function.'

The CUMULATIVE effect of smart, effective training can have some unexpected benefits. ☺

9

PUTTING IT ALL TOGETHER

A Different Resolution

Hoping you have a fantastic year! Reading this aloud to yourself for 21 days straight might be a Positive Difference maker... #AllTheBest

I will FINALLY open my mind to the reality all around me that I do not see. Regarding my health, I will commit to 1st understanding & then Believing that my broken body can & will Heal. It's not about the injured joints or the damaged muscles or the failing organs like my heart & lungs or my faulty metabolism that keeps me fat or some auto-immune dysfunction. It's not even about my Nervous System which controls & regulates everything.

It's ALL about what controls my nervous system. It's all about my Mind- what I know, what I believe, the habits I have allowed, the attitudes I have cultivated.

If I focus on my Mind, everything else will fall into place. But for most of us this will take time. It's not just about learning a new technique but more about having a revised Code to live by. And much will have to be un-learned.

The cumulative effect will be nothing short of miraculous. I have a plan to accomplish this. Most will fight this idea because they are overwhelmed with 'life' & would rather escape- through alcohol & drug use, techno-gadgetry, idle gossip, mindless exercise and over-eating.

Doing these things to escape will speed up my demise. I choose to 'turn on' my mind in order to continue growing. As we see in Nature all around us, when growth stops the dying begins.

MuscleByRussell

Resolutions Fail, Goals Succeed

I am reminded of the great Olympian Dan O'Brien.

As the 1991 World Decathlon Champion, O'Brien entered the Olympic year of 1992 as the favorite to win the gold medal at the 1992 Summer Olympics in Barcelona. The Olympic Gold Medal Decathlon Champion is considered the World's Greatest Athlete.

However, during the U.S. Olympic Trials O'Brien had a disaster in the 8th event- the Pole Vault. He failed to clear the bar on all three attempts. As a result, he scored no points and dropped from first place to 12th place among the 24 decathletes. He did not make the Olympic team for Barcelona, but he continued to train.

O'Brien's 'no height' in the pole vault was also a financial embarrassment for his main corporate sponsor, and for NBC television which was heavily promoting the upcoming Olympics. O'Brien appeared with U.S. rival Dave Johnson in the memorable Dan & Dave TV commercials for Reebok. The ads were meant to build interest in Reebok and the decathletes, culminating in the Olympics in Barcelona.

Dan's unexpected failure in the US Trials received considerable attention; Reebok adjusted by running new ads featuring him cheering on Dave who went on to win the bronze medal.

Even though he missed the Olympics, Dan went out later that summer and set the All Time Decathlon record in a competition in France… but he knew he would have to do it in the Olympics to be considered the all time great.

So he trained every day for the next 4 years and won the Gold Medal at the 1996 Olympic Games in Atlanta.

But here's the important part of the story for you. The 1st person Dan O'Brien thanked after winning Gold was a guy named Milt Campbell. Milt Campbell was the 1956 Olympic Decathlon Champion and the greatest all around athlete the state of New Jersey has ever produced.

After his bitter defeat in 1992, Dan was at a seminar and Milt Campbell was a guest speaker. Milt asked the question- 'Who here has a goal?' and Dan raised his hand.

Then Milt asked the next question- 'Who here has a goal and has it written down?'. Dan again raised his hand knowing that his goals were on a piece of paper somewhere in a drawer in his desk.

The final question was posed- 'Who here has a goal, has it written down and has it with them right now?' Milt pulled a neatly folded piece of paper out of his pocket. Dan did not raise his hand.

Milt believed that if you did not carry your goals with you at ALL times, you would get distracted and lose your focus. And that distractions and loss of focus were the key reasons that we all fail to achieve what we truly desire.

So there you have it. A practical plan anyone can follow. Set a goal and if you really want it, it will be yours. Goals help us reach our Dreams. A weak resolution might show us what we say we really want is just fantasy.

Over the years I have had to add 1 more piece to Milt Campbell's plan. Answer the question 'Who are you?' and have that at the top of the paper. During the times that you might feel defeated or worthless, it's important to remember how special you really are!

Get in Shape... WHY???

I'm going to be 66 this year and I've been working out for 45 years. I've been training people for 34 years. And while there are a few SECRETS to eating and training right, it surely is NOT nuclear physics.

You all KNOW the tremendous benefits of sound nutrition and regular exercise for you and your entire family. Then why the heck are we a country full of mostly fat, sick and poorly conditioned people?

A big part of the answer comes from a book my oldest daughter gave me for Christmas a few years back. It's probably not part of any course she's taking in college since it talks about what it means to be a man and what it means to be a woman. This seems to be a touchy subject in our culture and the writer puts it in your face, pulling no punches.

He contends that deep in his heart, every man longs for a BATTLE TO FIGHT, an ADVENTURE TO LIVE and a BEAUTY TO RESCUE. And the longing of the woman is equally exciting as the Great Adventure is SHARED.

I'll bet that if you had a big reason to REALLY LIVE, then training and eating right to get in shape would have some URGENCY. If you had some BIG DREAMS to chase, you would need your health to be at its optimal.

It's okay to be angry if you've allowed yourself to get swallowed up in a way of life that has sapped your strength and robbed your vitality. Don't make any 'doomed to fail' resolutions or excuses. Develop new HABITS. CHANGE your ATTITUDE and CHANGE the way you THINK… AND you'll end up in the best shape of your life- Physically, Mentally and Spiritually!!!

I'm always asked about the BEST exercise to do for troubling body parts. The BEST exercise we can do is to stop and THINK first. See where you are and what direction you should take.

It's been well said, 'Things which matter most, must never be at the mercy of things which matter least.'

This Wheel is a very powerful tool for working toward a more Balanced Life. I've utilized it in many different settings and the response has always been very appreciative.

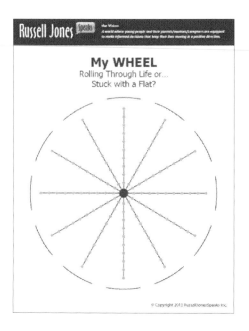

The Personal Growth & Development Wheel will take a few moments of quiet reflection and will lead you through 3 stages- Awareness, Decision, and On the Road. Once you become Aware of where you are right now, you will be able to make a Decision to make positive changes that will put you On the Road to a more balanced and fulfilled life.

Plan out some quiet time alone or with your spouse or trusted friend. As you go through this exercise, recognize the strength of a 3-legged stool and consider your responses with a Mind-Body-Spirit mindset.

Now it's time to label the spokes on your wheel. The following are the labels for my spokes that you are free to use or you can substitute with things that you value. I've got 12 spokes but you can use as many or as few as you need. The 12 are:

⇒ Family

⇒ Family Values-Spiritual

⇒ Social

⇒ Personal Fitness

⇒ Nutrition

⇒ Helping Others

⇒ Attitude

⇒ Self-Knowledge

⇒ Finances

⇒ Control Media Influence

⇒ 'Act As If'

⇒ Vocab

Okay, now we go around the Wheel and ask ourselves where we stand on each thing that we value. As we do this exercise, we'll rate ourselves on a scale of 0-10 and mark that place on the appropriate spoke. 0 is the hub and 10 is the outermost point. Here are some questions I asked myself:

Family- Define your family. How much do you value these relationships? Do you need to set aside 1 on 1 time especially with your spouse and children? If you're coming out of a dysfunctional family experience, is it time to do some work and come up with a 'model' to work toward?

Family Values-Spiritual- Are you where you want to be with the Creator of the Universe? Is your spirituality part of your lifestyle? Do you need to commit more time to prepare for eternity?

Social- Most people spend more time planning their vacations than they invest planning their lives. Does this fit you? Do you think all day about making it to 'happy hour'? What's more important- your career or your play time? Friends, vacations, and fun are important but…

Personal Fitness- Do you have a regular fitness routine? Does it include strength training, flexibility work, and conditioning? For optimal fitness and longevity, research shows that burning 2,000- 3,000 calories/ week through exercise is best- where do you stand? A gym membership is not required for optimal health and a sculpted body.

Nutrition- Do you have an overall philosophy when it comes to your diet? Do you understand the language- complete protein sources, simple vs. complex carbohydrates, good fats/ bad fats, natural vs. processed, flavor enhancers, artificial colors/ flavors, preservatives, etc.? Do you take supplements? Do you understand the process used to make supplements? 'All nutritional supplements are not created equal'. In terms of long-term health, it's been said that 'genetics loads the gun but lifestyle pulls the trigger'. How are you feeding the only body you will ever have for this lifetime?

Helping Others- A quote that we had on our refrigerator for years read as follows: 'The Secret of Happiness- Find a Hurt and Heal It!'. Do you set aside time to help others? It can be as a volunteer to care for the young, the elderly, the sick, the incarcerated, or the homeless. The ROI (return on investment) is tremendous. Get out of your little world and encourage someone else in theirs.

Attitude- Another famous quote states that 'your attitude will determine your altitude' in life. Are you an optimist or a pessimist? Positive or negative? You can change your life by changing your attitude. You can refuse to be negative. Utilize positive affirmations and positive self-talk. On this one, you might need to check with someone else about your attitude. The reason to check? Pigs don't know that pigs stink. Of course, this is coming from a former pig that had friends who helped him through the journey from extremely negative to positive.

Self-Knowledge- Many of us get to an age when 'adult' is stamped on our foreheads and we stop learning. One area that gets ignored is self-knowledge. Are you still growing? Do you have a system in place? How about reading for 15 minutes before bed every night in the 'classics'? Some of my favorite 'classics' include 'How To Win Friends & Influence People', 'The Power of Positive Thinking', & 'Psycho-Cybernetics'. If you can do it for 21 nights in a row, a fantastic habit will be yours. The biggest room in the world is the 'room for self-improvement'.

Finances- Some people love this stuff, others loathe it. Either way, do you have a plan? Are you where you want to be? Do you need counseling in this area? Another quote from the deep recesses of my brain- 'If you fail to plan, you automatically plan to fail'.

Control Media Influence- Some believe that they can watch or listen to all the violence and immorality they want. They believe that as long as something is not physically touching them, then it's okay. Others believe that who you are is predicated on your experiences. The acronym GIGO (garbage in, garbage out) probably applies here. Another way to look at it is to consider whether you believe that a person becomes like the people that he/she associates with. Do people who hang with violent, immoral people become like them? What effect will this have on you long-term? Does viewing violence and immorality over and over and over again make a person more tolerant about violence and immorality? Check what you're letting in your head- TV, movies, music, newspapers, magazines, etc.

'Act As If'- If you're not on the right track with your life, what else can you do? A friend of mine Dr. Rob Gilbert introduced me to 'Act As If' a long time ago. If you're not where you want to be as a student, in your career, in your business, in your relationships, then you might want to consider this powerful exercise. It's not something you do your whole life but for many of us 'Act As If' is very profitable for a season. Give your ego some time off and find someone who is where you want to be in life and do what they do. I applied this years ago in college and ended up graduating with honors. What did I do? I came prepared for class. I sat in the front. I sat up straight. I looked awake. I participated in class. I asked questions. I did

neat work. I handed in my assignments on time. I helped others. And I had a great attitude. Simple but not easy. Do you need to apply 'Act As If' in your life?

Vocab- Not just an exercise but a tool you can use to better yourself in many areas. The kids still call it vocab but I'm talking about vocabulary. Your ability to communicate and to understand is many times limited by your grasp of the English language. Many of us were short-changed in school and at home when we weren't challenged to increase our Word Power. Here's a simple exercise that greatly increased my vocabulary. For 3 years I carried a dictionary with me everywhere I went. I was pretty good at spelling and maybe using a word in a sentence but that wasn't good enough. If I could not clearly define a word, I would stop and look it up. In the beginning this was a major pain as I struggled through sentences. However, the results were phenomenal. How is your vocab? Do you need to get after it for a season?

The final step is to now connect the dots. Will your wheel roll? If it's anything like mine looked, it resembled a wheel you might see in the Flintstones. The Wheel will probably confirm your strengths and illuminate the areas that need work. Put an action plan together to round out your wheel. Nail this chart on your refrigerator as a reminder.

After a few months you'll be 'Rolling Through Life' instead of 'Stuck with a Flat'!

How I overcome Depression, Anxiety, Sadness, Frustration, Fear, Insecurity and a Bad Attitude

Life is hard-- really hard-- for everyone. And then every once in a while we get hit with something so bad we think we'll never survive it.

Probably my worst nightmare was a number of years ago when one of my sons was killed in a car crash. At one point I was so low that they put me on medication. That lasted one day. I got worse.

I learned that answers & solutions to life's big hits are not in a pill. *Medication never gets to the* **source** *of the pain.*

My solution has served me well for over 30 years now. It's based on my personal experience & has nothing to do with anyone's scientific studies or theories.

As I had to do, you must 'own your stuff'. And conquer it yourself. I know it will work because if I can do it- so can you.

Daily Check List for a Better Life:

Make your bed-

Accomplish the 1st task of the day. If you can't get the little things right, you'll never get the big ones right. I got this from a US Navy SEALs Admiral.

Read one chapter from the Book of Psalms Out Loud-

Please skip this one if you're not a believer. It not about religion, really. We all need to hear the Wisdom of the Ages. *I can't tell you how mad at God I was after my son died.*

Read one section of the New Testament Out Loud-

Please skip this one if you're not a believer. Getting insight into what Jesus was all about will at least help you understand your crazed Christian friends. And he was called the Prince of Peace & Peace is something we all need.

Breathe-

Deep, intentional, focused breathing rejuvenates every cell in your being. I like Wim Hof's method. It's quick & effective. 30 quick deep breaths without a full exhale. Empty yourself of air & stay empty as long as you can. Inhale one big breath & hold as long as you can. Repeat the entire cycle 2 more times.

Cold water rinse off-

This is my wimpy version of all the ice bath & cryogenics that is popular. At the end of a nice hot shower, turn the pressure down low and turn the temp down to cold. Let the water run over you (I have it aimed at my chest) for 15 seconds, build up to 1 minute. You will have an awesome glow for at least an hour afterward. I hate being cold. The effects of this are just the opposite. The process is counter-intuitive but very effective.

Read one chapter of a real book-

Get something that will Inspire or Motivate or Instruct you. Hold it in your hands. Don't rush through it. Pause and think about things. Underline what jumps out at you. Even if you only read 1 sentence that is profound, it can brighten your entire day.

Affirm positive things-

On a small piece of paper write down your goals. Also, write down the answer to the question 'Who are you?' Carry that piece of paper with you- everywhere. *Whenever your thinking gets dark or you feel defeated, read what is on the paper.* Use it as often as needed. Don't leave home without it.

Love on people instead of judging them-

This might be the hardest thing on the list. Fight to get it right as often as you can.

Get the blood pumping at least 3 times a day-

Even if you plan to work out later in the day or have already trained early, movement is vital through the entire day. 5-7 minutes 3 times a day is fine as long as it's done intelligently. Not only does it get your blood pumping to all your joints & work against the negative effects of sitting for long periods, it lifts your mood. There are movements one can do without any props or equipment that are very effective.

Eat smart-

Don't be a victim of processed foods or familial eating habits. The foods you eat can either add to your health & sense of well being or take away from it. A body that has to work overtime to digest is a stressed out body. Eat to nourish, repair and energize. Don't let old habits ruin your health and add to life's regular problems. If you think you know how to eat but are in terrible shape or have to be on medications then 'you really don't have a clue'.

Humble yourself. It's okay to need help. Seek out someone who exudes health & wellness not some 'expert' who does not look like they are taking their own advice. An older person would be a better choice here since the cumulative effect of what they believe will be visible. Be open to wisdom in this area.

Drink smarter-

Keep it pure. No sugar, no artificial sweeteners or flavorings or colorings. Be aware of how one becomes dehydrated. Dehydration makes the body feel stiff, de-energized and sluggish.

It's easy to stay hydrated.

My personal pet peeve- folks who walk around with a huge jug of water. Drink when you are thirsty. Too much water flushes out valuable minerals.

We all know the saying 'an apple a day keeps the doctor away'. Actually an apple a day (or 2 if you drink dehydrating beverages) is a much more efficient and healthful way to stay hydrated.

Put something positive in your head just before you shut the light out at night-

This is critical since your subconscious mind never sleeps. It keeps working. Giving it something positive & uplifting to work on through the night will yield a higher quality sleep.

Maybe it's that book you are reading or a quote from a favorite author or a prayer or a poem.

Try it out. Watch a scary movie followed by the day's news and go to sleep one night. Then see how you feel in the morning. The next night try my suggestion.

Don't leave this off your checklist.

Please note that this is a serious list. I am not trivializing serious mental conditions. *It has been my experience that in all medical matters a holistic approach always yields better results.*

Everything in the human body is connected. Unless it is blunt force trauma, I have found that where you feel hurt is not the origin or source of your pain.

Following this Daily Check List will help you to better 'own your health'. You will be empowered, strengthened and girded up. You will not get sick as often and if you do get sick or injured, you will recover faster.

Once you have taken command of yourself then you can enjoy true happiness. For to have true happiness we must be strong enough to reach beyond ourselves. It's been posted on each refrigerator I've had for the last 35 years- The Secret of Happiness? Find a Hurt & Heal It.

Get outside yourself and really live.

As my old friend David DeNotaris always says- Make It a Great Day!....

10

Russell's True Health Care Bill

Okay,okay,okay (say it really fast like Leo Getz in Lethal Weapon2) help me here. The government is taking over Health Care in the United States.

First of all, there never was Health Care in the United States only Sick Care. And Sick Care is needed and we need a lot of it. 'Preventative medicine' is just a buzzword for 'testing to see if you are Sick yet'.

WE THE PEOPLE have brought this on ourselves through ignorance and laziness. My Mother taught me a long time ago that we have to be proactively in charge of our own health. The early 'health food nuts' and 'fitness crazies' were Right. But we all have to come to grips with the fact that none of us are getting out of here alive.

We have to realize a few things:

1. The majority of 'foods' on the shelf in our grocery stores are g-a-r-b-a-g-e. It's legal but it shouldn't be. Most food

processing companies are driven by 1 thing and that is Profit (for themselves and you who hold stock). As has been pointed out many times before---- if whatever you are buying has Sugar in any of its forms, White Flour or Chemical Additives, you are setting yourself and your family up for sickness, disease and pre-mature death.

2. Most Doctors DO know their *ss from their elbow- and that's a good thing. However, 99.9% of the doctors we come across Specialize in something other than nutrition. Yet many dispense nutritional opinions and most of us buy their opinions.

    And the Nutritionists I've met are too concerned with counting Calories and the Fat content of foods that they miss the boat when it comes to Fresh, Wholesome Foods from a variety of Natural sources. And they do not have a handle on Natural Supplementation. Methinks they 'compromise' too much and need to raise the standards and expectations. Nutrition Experts need to get radical and scream out 'warnings' to our culture. Also, the food pyramid and its various versions have not worked.

3. Pharmaceutical Companies do not have a moral compass. The researchers might but Drug Companies

are driven by 1 thing and that is Profit (for themselves and you who hold stock). They are the best and worst of what big business is all about. They have had a huge hand in crafting our Drug Culture. They have pushed their 'miracle cures' on the medical community and on WE THE PEOPLE to a degree that is almost unfathomable.

Some of the stuff works but most are nonsense- the side effects alone are embarrassing.

4. Insurance Companies do not have a moral compass. I believe in free enterprise but Insurance Companies are so unscrupulous they NEED regulation. Insurance Companies are driven by 1 thing and that is Profit (for themselves and you who hold stock).

5. Government has a real hard time acting objectively when it comes to Most issues. Partisan politics has our elected officials voting the Party line. Lobbyists influence all levels of government and are only interested in furthering the interests of those who Pay them.

Someone has proposed that whatever the government gives us (We The People) in Health (Sick) Insurance would be what all elected officials would have to use as well.

6. Lawyers! They are so intertwined in all of the above that they can make a well person sick. And they would figure out a way that *it would be 'prejudicial and unjust' to treat someone who abuses their health any differently than someone who makes the effort to take care of themselves.* What?? That's just crazy talk!

So this is what I'm going to use to start Russell's True Health Care Bill. I'm borrowing it from my old friend Arthur Dreschler as he wrote in the November 2009 Association of Oldetime Barbell & Strongmen Newsletter:

'While there are many issues regarding the health of this nation's citizens, and that of people throughout the world, and change is going on all around us, at least one thing remains true. Progressive resistance exercise is one of the greatest discoveries in human history. It has the ability to heal the sick, strengthen the weak, inspire the downtrodden and transform the body and soul. Its benefits are available to all, without exception. And when such training is combined with sound dietary practices and abstinence from debilitating practices, such as the use of alcohol and drugs, a recipe for a longer and a more vigorous life is created. NOTHING MORE IS NEEDED, BUT NOTHING LESS IS SUFFICIENT.

... Nothing would benefit the health of the nation more quickly and completely, or reduce our health care costs more surely, then the widespread adoption of regular (ideally progressive) exercise, a sound diet and the avoidance of dissipation. Given this we should all redouble our efforts to extol the virtues of exercise and other sound health practices, while at the same time ASSURING THAT WE ARE EACH LIVING EXAMPLES OF WHAT WE ESPOUSE.'

Fight for YOUR Health!

Here then is just one response to my suggestion.

It was submitted by none other than Mr. Steve Perillo- Perillo Tours CEO- Mr. Italy Jr. Aside from running Perillo Tours and being an accomplished classical composer/recording artist, Steve also hosts his own talk show.

And while not being an unabashed 'health nut' like myself, Steve eats and supplements wisely AND he works out regularly.

He writes the following in response to Russell's True Health Care Bill:

HERE! HERE! Right on! Imagine exercise and diet credits! . . . like a 'good driver' getting lower insurance rates. 50% of all kids born today will get juvenile diabetes? Even if that's a huge exaggeration, 5% of kids getting that would be absurd.

Sorry to say, if you let market forces go wild, with no oversight, this is what we get . . . 150 pound, ten year olds playing video games all day while eating Coco-Puffs, unable to go outside because they need their parents to drive them everywhere. Our 'junk culture' is killing our children!

Sorry we're too stupid to oversee ourselves because now we need laws to force us to behave:

1. *Restrict amounts of sugar in products*

2. *No sugar at all in schools*

3. *Sidewalks and bike-lanes mandatory for all new suburban constructions*

4. *No school bussing if you live within 1 mile of school*

5. *Food stamps only good for certain food purchases*

6. *Stop farm subsidies (corn) that promote tons of cheap, hormone and antibiotic injested beef and poultry.*

The corporations don't care. Just the opposite. They're incentivized to create customer addictions!

They have multi-million dollar labs that study how to turn consumers into those lab rats . . . pawing the 'more cocaine button' until they kill themselves.

And what's addicting? Cheap fat, salt and carbs. And for some reason those are the cheapest materials to put on the table! (See corn subsidies!)

McDonalds is currently the cheapest way to feed a family of 4 . . . $12! Fruits and vegetables cost way more than that to feed the same family.

We used to be a lean, mean country . . . No mas!

Steve

Like me, Steve has an objective advantage over our lawmakers in Washington. He's not a lawyer who has been elected to public office. He's not 'beholding' to any self-serving lobby groups.

Don't shrug off this topic. Think it through and come up with YOUR Personal Wellness Plan. Remember- once your Body is weakened by all the drugs and junk food being pumped into it, YOUR Mental, Emotional and Spiritual Strength is sure to follow.

The so called 'greatest country in the history of the world', the country that has sacrificed many thousands of lives to keep our freedom and to save millions of people around the world, the land of the free and the home of the brave is SICK. The corrupt money gods are creating wealth for themselves but force-feeding us a steady diet of dead, nutrition-less foods just to fill our bellies.

The ENEMY is within and it ain't just a bunch of crazed terrorists. In the same way We The People have fought for our Freedom, we must fight for our HEALTH!

11

ABOUT ME

Well this is fantastic! I was named to a list of the 'Top 100-plus Strongest Coaches to Learn from in 2016 and Beyond- A Rebellion in Fitness'.

It's an international list and comes from the founder of An Unconventional Life- Bud Jeffries.

The criteria is awesome- *So – here are the qualifications to be on this list:*

They have to be legit, world-class strong in one way or another or have been at some time in their life if they are older and choosing to pursue lighter things now. There are many ways to be strong and not everyone here is going to be the same kind of strong. That's okay boys and girls, everyone doesn't have to do the same thing. We're not going to be strength fascists. They have to have proved this in one way or another – either via competition or video. This isn't the 1940s and we aren't accepting hear-say legends, because Uncle Bob swears he saw it happen. Every five-year-old on the planet has a camera phone so pics or video or it didn't happen.

Finally, they have to publicly teach or coach or produce information in some way that you can get your hands on to actually learn from them and it can't be plagiarized, repackaged information from someone who really IS strong.

The point here – This is an honest, organic list of true trainers who know what they're doing, not just looking to turn other people's insecurities and popular Google topics into a fast buck with slick marketing. These are men and women who have dedicated their time, study, effort and sweat into the world of strength and fitness, becoming exceptional at their craft and have chosen to then share that knowledge with others.

This is great because 10 years ago I thought it might be all over in regards to strength. The injuries were mounting and that was causing the motivation to wane. But it was my fortune to stumble upon a system of training that changed my life. I then tweaked it with a wise eating and supplementing regimen.

At almost 66 years old, I feel better than I did at 40. As I look around and see how most exercise is being done, I just shake my head.

When we're young we can do just about anything physical and get some kind of 'results'- usually drop a few pounds and get a very fleeting period of muscular hypertrophy aka 'beach muscle'. Unfortunately the 'pump' is usually not based on real strength. People get better at technique (or begin to cheat on their form) and their numbers (reps, sets & poundages) go up- - for a short period.

The truth is we as a culture are not patient enough or wise enough to understand this. That's why most fitness fanatics freak out if they have to take a lay off for sickness or any other reason. *True strength is not fleeting once it is attained.*

But mindless exercise leads to injury. Injury leads to the development of compensations. As we run out of compensations, we run to doctors and chiros and PTs and anyone we think can 'cure' us. Meds are added in along the way. And don't forget the braces, tapes and wraps.

We all know how so many aspects of life are corrupt- politics, business, science, education, religion, and on and on. Health and fitness are the same.

I love how folks come and tell about their physical ailments and weakness and how they are overweight and have no energy. And they tell me what they need to do but they don't. And they tell me how they 'used' to be in great shape and they want to get back to that.

But that's the problem really. They know so much they can't hear the truth or they can't accept the fact that they did it all wrong and they are afraid to 'start over'. But if they only took a little bit of time and became a student of how it should be done, they would be in fantastic shape. *Starting over is liberating!*

C'est la vie.

I truly love those who want to learn, who want to accomplish something great. Like young athletes or regular folks who want to live a vibrant life not restricted by physical ailments.

So thanks again to An Unconventional Life for this recognition. Sometimes you wonder if anyone is watching.

Age- 65, lifetime steroid & Performance Enhancing Drug free, no cosmetic enhancements

Signature Feat- June 7, 2008, on the occasion of the 25th anniversary of the Association of OldeTime Barbell & Strongmen's 1st gathering, Russell Jones attempted a feat of strength **NEVER TRIED BEFORE**.

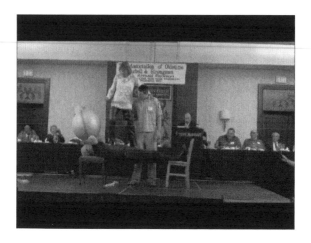

With his body suspended face-up between 2 chairs... And with his wife, Lin standing on his stomach... Russell blew up and burst a Hot Water Bottle with only lung power... The back pressure alone was incredible... it took between 500 and 700 pounds of pressure to get a **REAL** one to explode... <u>No mouthpieces or plugs were used</u>.

This is a **REAL** hot water bottle from the CARA Corporation, Warwick, RI, USA.

'As a witness it was very exciting and I was drawn into the extreme stress that Mr. Jones was forced to endure. As a Medical Professional I had grave concerns about the well-being of the performer. DO NOT try this one at home.'

Robert M. Goldman MD, PhD, DO, FAASP

Chairman of the Board-A4M

World Chairman-International Medical Commission

Chairman-World Academy of Anti-Aging Medicine

President Emeritus-National Academy of Sports Medicine

Guinness Book World Record Holder

Best Selling Author- **'Death in the Locker Room'**

Full length version available on request--
https://www.instagram.com/p/1se_QEp_2i/?taken-by=russelljonesspeaks

Some other strength feats

⇒ Blow up and burst a Hot Water Bottle... with lung power

⇒ Bend a 60 penny nail in half... with bare hands

⇒ Tear a deck of plastic coated playing cards in half with hands behind back. Tear the remaining halved deck into quarters... using only grip strength.

⇒ Demonstrate a human bridge... while performing incredible feats

⇒ Bend a ½″ thick, round steel bar... around the neck... into a fish!

⇒ Scrolling Steel Bars

⇒ Smash 9- 2″ thick bricks... with one crushing blow

⇒ Smash 8 1x12 boards no spacers

⇒ Nail Driving

⇒ Hold back 2 strong guys... with one hand

⇒ While suspended between 2 chairs with 2 cement blocks on stomach... have someone break the blocks with a huge sledge hammer

⇒ Roll up a frying pan into a tube

Association of Oldetime Barbell & Strongmen appearances- 4

Speaking & Coaching-

http://www.russelljonesspeaks.com/

Book- Top Secrets of Success... 4 Kids

http://www.russelljonesspeaks.com/top-secret-book.html

Base of Operations-

http://www.mybackandbodyclinic.com/

Experience-

Master Trainer - Muscle By Russell, 1984 - present

- ❖ A fitness training and consulting business

the PowerWorkshop, 1993 - present

- ❖ Over 1,000 speaking engagements on Motivation, Self-esteem and Health & Wellness.

Author- *'Top Secrets of Success… 4Kids'*

Author – Weekly Breakthrough Newsletter, 2005 - present

- ❖ Content available through website archive

NJ State Department of Education, 2003 - present

- ❖ Professional development provider

Functional Fitness Trail Design, 2002 Saddle River, NJ

- ❖ Innovative nature-friendly apparatus over a ½ mile course

Creator - Personal Growth & Development Breakthrough Wheel, 2005

- ❖ Powerful tool to evaluate strengths and weaknesses

Sources for Training Expertise

- ❖ Dennis Rogers - The Strongest Man in the World, pound for pound

- ❖ Jay Schroeder - Originator of the World's Best Training System- UltraFit EvoSport

- ❖ Denis Thompson - Founder of the Fastest System to Recover from Injury- ARPwave

Certifications

- ❖ NGA Certified Master Fitness Trainer -35 years

- ❖ ARPwave Neurological Strength Therapist - 12 years

- ❖ AOBS Professional Strength Athlete - 26 years

- ❖ NJ State Teaching Certification

- ❖ Healthcare Professional Certifications- BCLS: Adult CPR, Child CPR & Infant CPR, Emergency Basic First Aid, Cognitive A.E.D. Skills

Pulling from life changing experiences, I speak to the heart of issues that negatively affect personal drive and performance.

I only mention that I am 65 years old because '65 is the new 40'- at least for me!

In response to a series of health problems & injuries, I started my foray toward a healthy lifestyle. What I have discovered can help anyone get on the road to a Better Life.

I humbly learned from both experts and my own successes and failures. And now I'm sharing my deep experience on what has worked well. To weather any storms, I came up with anchor points and that will spark you to identify your own anchors. The cumulative effect of life-giving habits is truly awesome.

12

88 OTHER IMPORTANT THINGS TO PAUSE AND THINK ABOUT

#TeachYourChildren- Remembering a day at the Jersey Shore around 1989! My oldest daughter- what an AMAZING childhood she had!

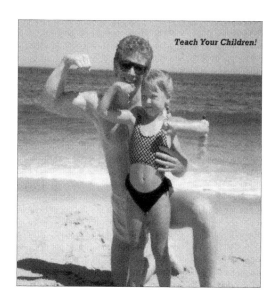

And now she's an AMAZING Woman!

Which way to the Beach? ☺

Another pic of the craziest thing I ever attempted. It looks like GrandMaster Strongman Dennis Rogers' head is sitting atop the Hot Water Bottle. ☺ And that's my youngest son (#RussBuddy) EXHORTING me not to give up...

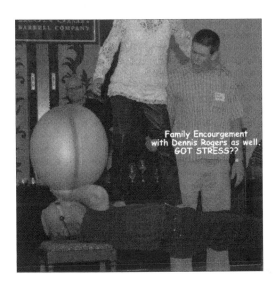

#Glad2Live2Tell

Teach Your Children Well!

She's 29 now & knows what the fitness lifestyle is all about. Teach it & Model it!

It's called passing along something of VALUE to your kids. ☺

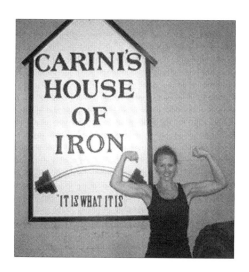

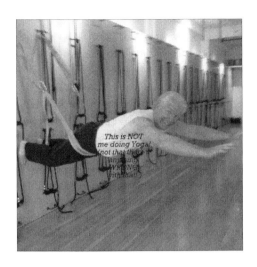

This is NOT me doing yoga! (not that there's anything WRONG with that). Actually this is a wall we will be building for our new My Back & Body Clinic here in New Jersey.

It looks like I'm posing as Superman but my instructor Jane Docampo from #janedocampobackcare and the owner of My Back and Body Clinic has me JUMPING on/off the wall in this position.

Methinks she wants to know if 62 year olds still have SPRING ☺. The answer is YES!

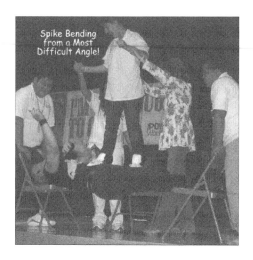

Bending a Spike the Hard Way!

When attempting to Bend, Break or Tear things, this position makes things quite difficult. Activating the Core along with the Hamstrings is essential... I never had Hammies until I turned 55.

So glad I learned how to train properly-- never2late ☺

1984ish original Muscle by Russell logo done by a girl named Mary...

32 years as a Trainer/Coach--- I'm thankful to be able to serve & help & guide & encourage...

The toughest part was sifting through all the 'total nonsense' being sold as HEALTHY—

be it Exercise, Food or Supplements...

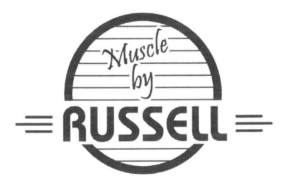

cardio ???corestrength ???Encouragement From GrandMaster Strongman Dennis Rogers.

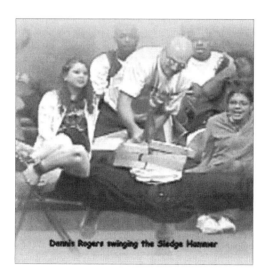

Dennis Rogers swinging the Sledge Hammer

Sledgehammer to Gut! (plz don't try this one at home Boys & Girls) ☺

In my Great GrandParent's kitchen was this piece of wrought iron that said- 'VE GET TOO SOON OLDT UNDT TOO LATE SCHMART'.

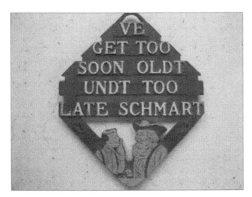

And there was an image of a wise older man giving some sage advice to a young man. The young man actually appeared Happy to receive what he was being told.

Pause & Think about THAT!! ☺

Old Guy Wannabe Gangsta!

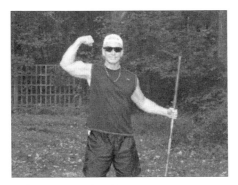

Snow on the Roof, Fire in the Furnace.

My Youngest Daughter-- not sure where she is going with this Beastly apparatus ☺ AND where is the HAPPY face?? LOL! @yogaonthecoast

I know people like to get all crazy during their workouts BUT sometimes you can get Mad Strong just by Holding Your Position... just sayin'.

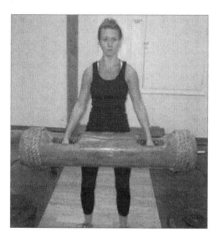

Watermelon Abs? My youngest son demonstrates how to train abs hard while activating the adductors...

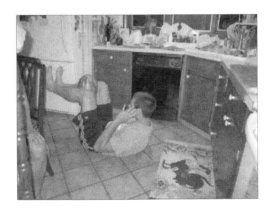

Of course he did it on the kitchen floor just before we all demanded that the Watermelon be sliced and properly devoured ☺

Breaking huge stacks of bricks, Blowing up thick Hot Water Bottles till they burst & having Concrete Blocks smashed on my stomach while suspended between 2 chairs--

YET it's not about me!

It's about the Message...& it's really all about YOU! That's why the audience is usually quite HAPPY.

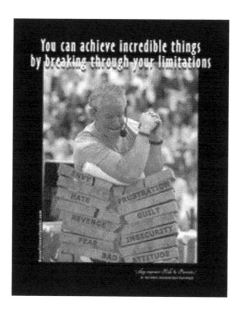

Doorway Chin Ups 1963 @ age 12

Getting ready to go for the Boy Scouts Personal Fitness Merit Badge! The badge was all the Motivation this young lad needed.

Thankful for the Fitness Foundation it provided!

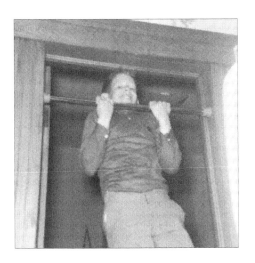

It was so cold I got goose bumps-- 2 Big Ones ☺ End of Winter Snow Workout ☺-- When Shoveling is just Not Enough - Age 61 but not done (yet-LOL)... Thanks to @yogaonthecoast for forcing me to post this!!

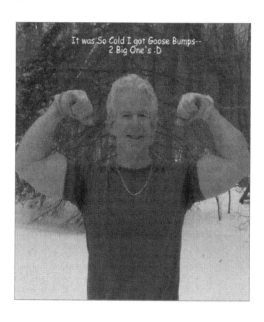

Deep Well Finger Tip Training! Be creative in where you exercise! Have fun doing Human movements!

Some think that in order to do a pull up, they need to use an official pull up bar located at an official pull up facility... This old WELL is a perfect example for this DEEP subject.

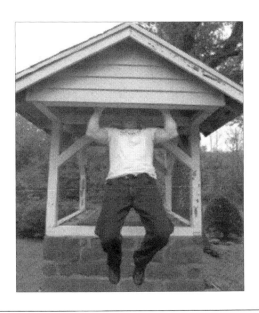

Vince Gironda Dip Bars I had made for a client when I designed his Fitness Trail back in the 90's... I make Dips a full body workout with a myriad of variations!

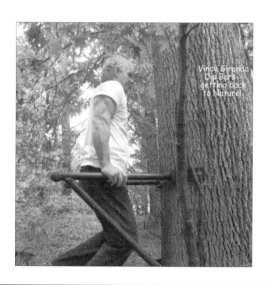

Car Lifting is a great workout if you can't get to the gym... this is my GreatGrandma's 1956 Dodge that I bought from her in the 1970s-- YIKES! If cars could tell stories.

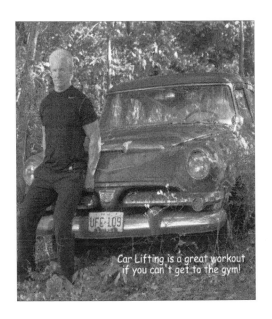

1979 Happy Painter! Today's workout IS painting-- ugh-- Attitude Check! ☺ Fear the Fro! LOL!

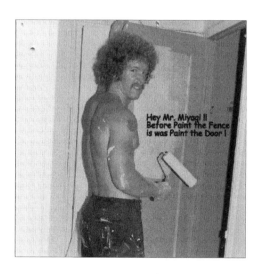

Curls for the Girls!! Even @ age 61?? LOL WhyNOT?

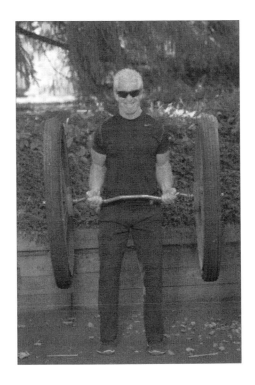

Freaky Forearm posedown with Ms. Olympia Carla Dunlap. A very gracious lady I met at the Association of Oldetime Barbell & Strongmen's annual banquet. That rare combination of Strength & Classic Beauty...

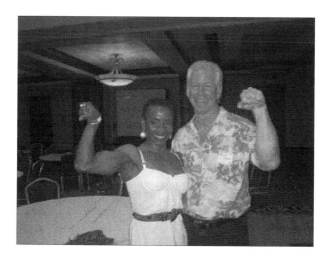

Scrolling a heavy metal bar into a piece of exercise equipment-- a Pec Pumper! *A professional strength athlete or Strongman is not a magician or performer of tricks. The feats are real and some are downright dangerous. But throughout history, real strength has had a place of honor in cultures around the world. Even the most sophisticated of audiences seem to get drawn into the awesome struggle and then victory in attempting what would appear to be an impossible task.* After a serious scroll of a heavy Steel Bar--- the special effect my friend put on is a tad Creepy! ☺

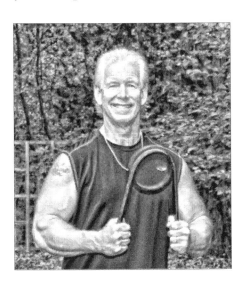

GrandMaster Strongman Dennis Rogers NOT tearing my arm off!!! tytyty Actually Arm Wrestling is a fantastic activity for raising Testosterone production which is important for those of us who want to go through this life ALL Natural...After nearly 62 years on this planet, I'm not buying into the 'science' that says I can't produce enough of my own hormones as I get older. Thankfully I've been around folks who believe the same.

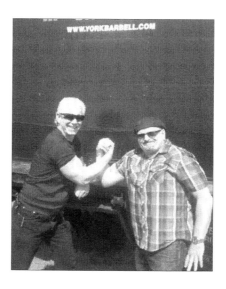

Happy college prof after tearing a deck of playing cards in half! It took a lot of screaming & yelling to keep him motivated even though he's a Sport Psychologist. Had to get him past the pain in his hands & the negative message 'I can't do this' swirling in his head--- but it had a Happy Ending. ☺

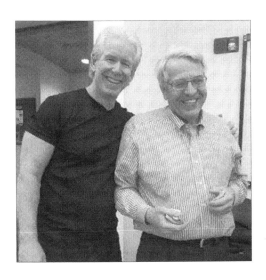

We ALL have times when we feel helpless & small & insignificant... ride it out by remembering who you really are & WHY you're on this Planet!!

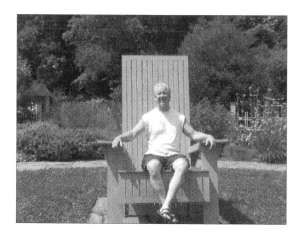

This was my Grandpa Jones' wheelbarrow from 1953! He got it the year I was born!

Some of my friends lift big stones for a great workout-- I did it because we had to dig a trench for our swimming pool!

So many people get crazy if they don't work out in a gym & do their routine... Methinks that there are a myriad of ways to exercise my body and if I miss a day with the 'official' weights at an 'authentic' gym-- so what? When you get too rigid about your training you burn out on a lot of levels & progress comes to a screeching halt!

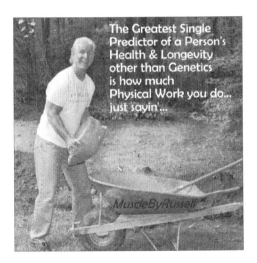

The Greatest Single Predictor of a Person's Health & Longevity other than Genetics is how much Physical Work you do... just sayin'...

Garden Planting in North Carolina! My Momma needed some help!

Tomatoes, Cukes, Beans, Lettuce--- ALL from Organic, Non-GMO seeds- YAY!

It this fast-paced world Gardening really forces us to slow down. No matter how amped up we are to 'get things done', we have to wait for the Seed to do its thing.

Lessons in Patience, Hope, & Nurturing all wrapped up in a little seed. It reminds me of that famous song 'Only two things that money can't buy >That's true love and home grown tomatoes'!

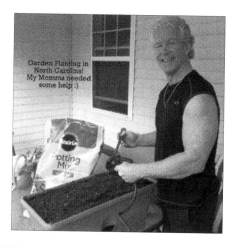

Too Tough To Quit-- from the back of my original 1987 TShirt when I went full time in Fitness Training/Coaching. I also used the quote in my book Top Secrets of Success... 4 Kids in the Dreambuilding/ GoalSetting section...

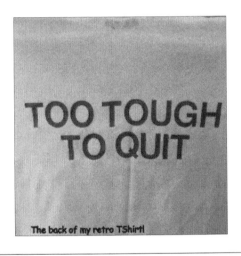

The back of my retro TShirt!

I'm calling this pic of me the UggLee Mug. ☺ So grateful that I was able to heal fast from surgery & return to 'better than ever' shape! Just looking at this pitiful face HAS to give you HOPE!

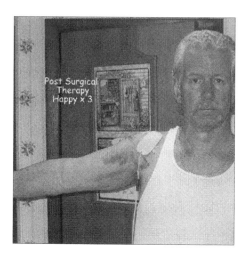

Afternoon Workout hoisting a few wheels I found on the old farm across the street. BUT I needed more Resistance! (never say 'I needed to add more WEIGHT' when lifting a Woman!!)

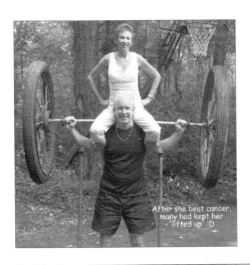

Philly is a tough place! They even have fight clubs in their churches! This is Pastor Jamie from In the Light Church. Aside from me breaking & bending a few things for the large group of men assembled, they had an actual ring set up with MMA fighters going at it! Talk about a scary amount of testosterone being generated. ☺ All joking aside... a great group of guys trying to do things right!

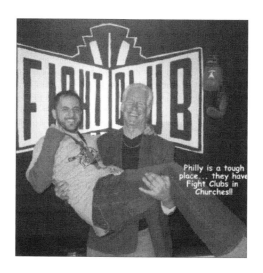

They broke but did not fall! Over the years I have probably smashed at least 800 stacks of bricks during my presentations. I call the 9 2" thick bricks the Wall of Negative and have names for all the bricks-- fear, bad attitude, laziness etc. Well a few years back at a corporate gig, I hit them hard enough to break but not hard enough to fall-- Inconceivable!!!

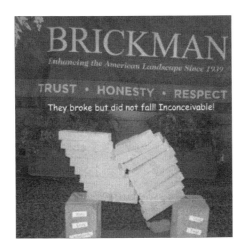

With the only 2 GrandMaster Strongmen on this Planet... Slim the Hammerman & Dennis Rogers!! Let's hear it for the Ol' Guys!!!

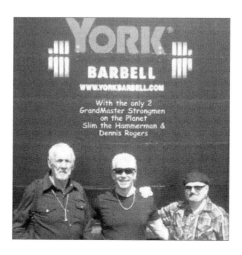

I see all kinds of delicious looking meals posted everywhere. But sometimes I'm in a Big HURRY and need something fast!

So I know what I do & don't eat & I hate to compromise so----

A handful of TJoes Sweet Potato chips crushed, a huge dollop of TJoes unsalted Almond Butter, a large scoop of Dennis Roger's Protein Powder & 5 drops of Organic Maple syrup...

Take a spoonful in your mouth with a sip of well water-- mix, chew, swallow, repeat

So I repeat the ??? Would YOU eat like this??

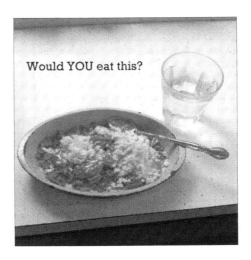

Would YOU eat this? Part2

I see all kinds of delicious looking meals posted everywhere. But sometimes I'm in a Big HURRY and need something fast!

So I know what I do & don't eat & I hate to compromise so----

Quickly chop up some Trader Joe's Cukes, scramble 3 large eggs from my neighbor's henhouse in a mix of Organic Coconut Oil & Olive Oil then lay it over a 1/2 teaspoon of Minerals (very salty taste)... add some fresh pepper---

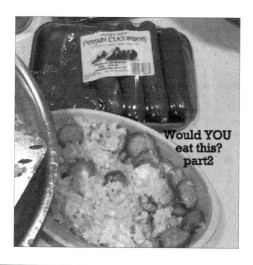

Would YOU eat this? Part3

I worked out with 1 of my Gorilla sons this morning... & by 4pm I was HUNGRY! Not usually a mealtime but I needed to EAT.

And I was in a HURRY!

1 can tJoe's unsalted Tuna, 2 dollops of Avocado Oil MAYO, a leftover cooked2perfection Sweet Potato, Pepper & Pink Salt... Yum ☺

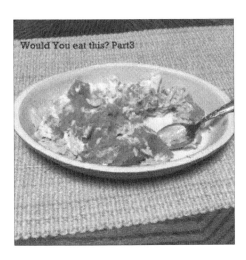

In Slim the Hammerman's Gym, Grandmaster Strongman Dennis Rogers, the Irish Anvil, Greg Matonick & me. A Joyful bunch of Mugs if there ever was!!! LOL!!!!

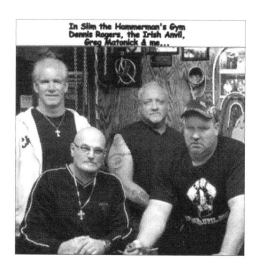

Got Jones? Travelling the High Road!

-- last minute T-shirt designed by Big Sister.

On the way to the NJ State Wrestling Championships 2009. What a year that was!!!

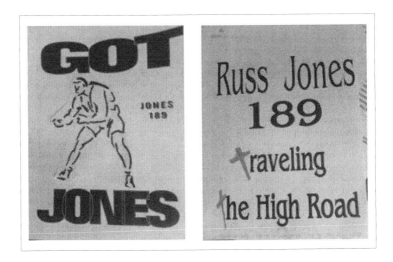

1993-- After just 1 Week of Exercise! Of course I'm just joking about 'after just 1 week'. But think about all the ads we see that make totally ridiculous claims- lose 100 pounds in 100 hours and all the altered before & after pics we can't help but look at.

If a person truly wraps there head around the meaning of the word CUMULATIVE, attaining whatever health or fitness goals they may have is well within reach.

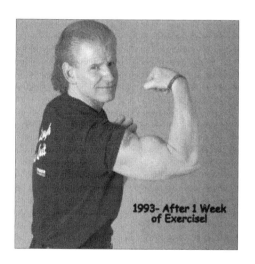

1993- After 1 Week of Exercise!

Being interrogated in a church in Chinatown, New York City! They wanted me to swear I was telling the TRUTH! I had a chance to speak to a group of teens & young adults. This picture was part of the evening. Great Kids & even greater Leaders... AND the Food was legend. I never knew folks actually ate carp!

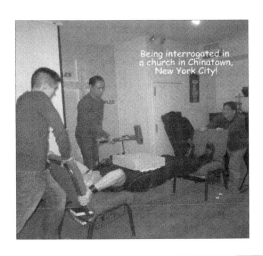

1994

I had been a performing Strongman for about 2 years and I was poor. How poor?

I was So poor I had to use my kids as Barbells!!! (not Dumbbells)

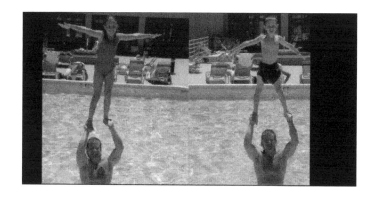

I only have about a month b4 my 62 bDay... hoping to represent. Morning Workout hoisting a few wheels I found on the old farm across the street. Make your training FUN but never compromise POSITION!

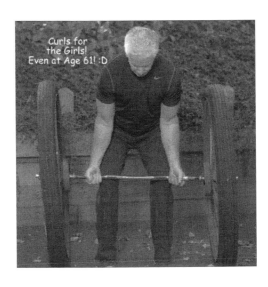

Happy St. Patrick's Day from the son of a shanty Irish lass. ☺
Now if I could just lift these 2 in 10 years-- THAT would be a
feat! Love the Grands!

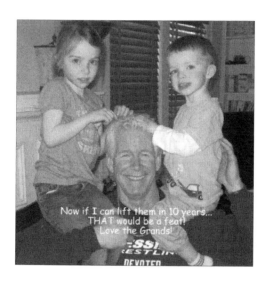

Driving a Nail through a thick Board with 1 punch! Dennis Rogers taught this to me many years ago... the balloon is under the board so the audience can see that it goes through. I would have someone in the audience come up to try & pull the nail out--- which they could never do. The Message? 'It's a lot easier to do something, than it is to try to undo something' Pause & think about that.

Warning-- Do NOT try this at home! If the nail does not go through the board, it can end up going through Your Hand. 😨

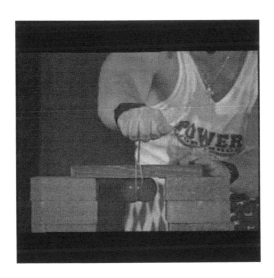

Practicing some new stuff--- in SloMo!!! 6 boards, no spacers, 4 5/8" thick-- will do 8 when I take the Show on the Road. Even @ age 61 setting new goals keeps things FRESH!

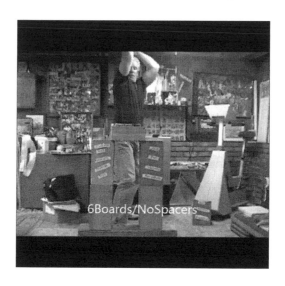

In the strongman world, taking and bending a heavy steel bar like this is called 'Scrolling'. I call it 'painful'. It's a pretty cool feat because each bend gets more difficult as you progress... & if you slow down to catch your breath the steel begins to harden as it cools-- motivation to keep moving 4sure. ☺

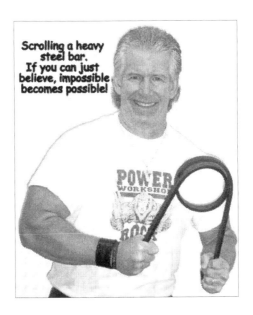

Scrolling a heavy steel bar. If you can just believe, impossible becomes possible!

Holding 4 lovely & strong ladies-- with 1 hand!!! There are many hidden messages one might derive from this video-- suffice to say it was fun!!

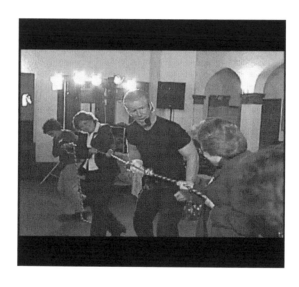

Spike Bending 101-- this is usually the 1st feat newbies must master. My teacher Dennis Rogers 'insisted' I use small pieces of washrags to protect my skin. I cried real tears until callous was built up in the right places. I think Dennis thought of it as De-Sensitivity Training!

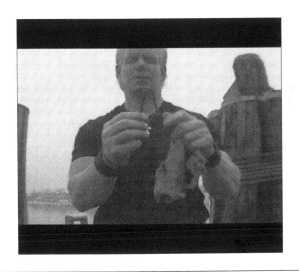

Do you trust your friends?? Here I'm holding a thick block of wood. GrandMaster Strongman Dennis Rogers lights a flammable liquid on Fire as I hold tight (eyes closed). He then drives a big Nail through the board with 1 punch. His arm moved so fast that it blew out the Flames!!!

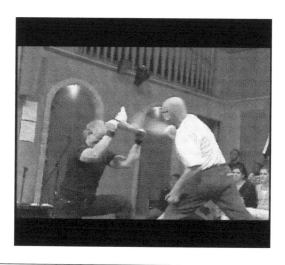

Happy St. Patrick's Day from the son of a shanty Irish lass. ☺

Tearing a new deck of Bicycle playing cards-- Behind the Back!

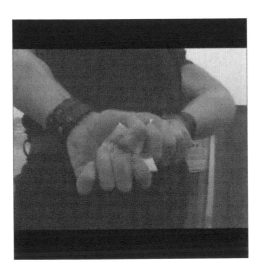

The Vision- A world where all people are equipped to make informed decisions that keep their lives moving in a positive direction. Using the experience of others is Wise.

FYI- I'm Bending a short 1/2" thick round steel bar around my neck... into a FISH! White Hair does NOT mean weak!

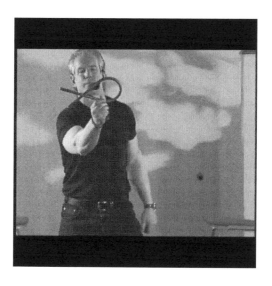

Lord, please let me be the person my Dog thinks I am! That is Rev the Therapy Dog-- 10 year old American Bulldog>> wait till you hear how he went from fat to jacked-- truStory!

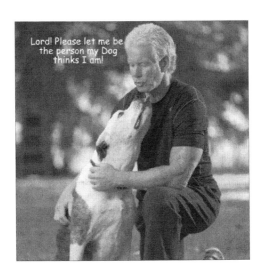

Asthma & Allergies can be CURED! Blowing up & bursting a real Hot Water Bottle- it takes between 500 & 700 pounds of pressure to do it! Not bad for a kid who HAD severe Asthma and Allergies! Thanks to my Mom who cleaned up my diet & gave me the right supplements!

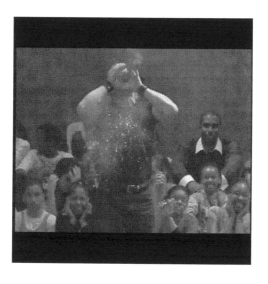

Rolling Up a Frying Pan into a Burrito Maker!!!

Not the tightest roll but my excuse is that it was freezing cold & the pan was frozen.

BUT I KNOW, I know 'NO EXCUSES'.

Thanks to my mentor GrandMaster Strongman Dennis Rogers--- I'm able to have FUN @ age 62 doing INSANE things!

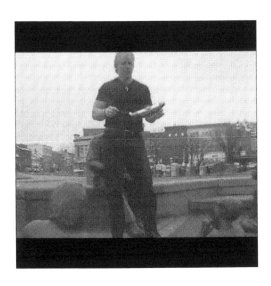

I hope you and your family have seen the Academy Award winning movie-'Chariots of Fire'. I didn't really 'get it' the first time I saw it but Chariots of Fire is very powerful. There's a scene at Cambridge University in which the head of the school summarizes what sport should be.

'Here... we've always been proud of our athletic prowess. ...we've always believed that our games are Indispensable in helping to complete... a person's Education. They create Character. They foster Courage and Leadership. But most of all an unassailable spirit of Loyalty, Comradeship, and Mutual Responsibility.' Would you agree?

So then the quote from Eric Liddell in the movie is this---

"In the dust of defeat as well as the laurels of victory, there is glory to be found if one has done his best."

Is this what kids today take away from their experiences in sport?

There is a sacredness in tears. They are not the mark of weakness, but of power. They speak more eloquently than ten thousand tongues. They are the messengers of overwhelming grief, of deep contrition, and of unspeakable love.

- Washington Irving

The legendary behavioral scientist William James put it this way IF YOU WANT TO CHANGE some of YOUR stinkin', no-good, life-shortening, makin'-you-uglier-than-you-really-are dirty-rotten' HABITS:

1. START IMMEDIATELY!

2. DO IT FLAMBOYANTLY!!

3. NO EXCEPTIONS!!!

In the office at Camp Marcella for the Visually Impaired in New Jersey I saw this quote on the wall--

If you want to be happy for an hour… go watch TV.

If you want to be happy for a day… go to an amusement park.

If you want to be happy for a LIFETIME… GO OUT & HELP OTHERS!

'A mirror can't change you; it can only let you know that YOU NEED TO CHANGE' –RJ

If you're reading this, YOUR ASSIGNMENT for today is get out of your comfort zone, your lazy place. ENCOURAGE A KID. Yes, even the one that you look at and cringe. The freakazoids and the gangsta wannabes and the too shy to look at you and all the ones that you think 'if they were my kid, I'd straighten them out in a hurry'. EMBRACE THEIR IDIOSYNCRACIES AND GIVE THEM A WORD OF ENCOURAGEMENT. No judgment. Just SOW some good seed INTO a YOUNG PERSON (if you have any extra---grown-ups could use some too). Keep GIVING (thanks). YOU WON'T BE DISAPPOINTED. -RJ

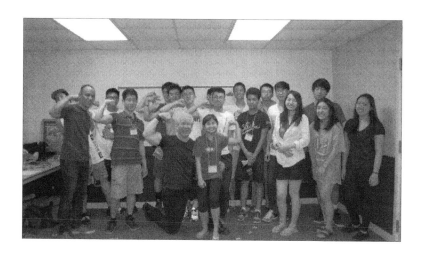

Fact of Life Department: 'Properly Raising a Teenager is like Trying to Nail Jell-O to a Tree!'

Question to Ask Yourself Department: 'Both enthusiasm and pessimism are contagious. How much of each do you spread???' -RJ

'I have Love in my Heart even though I have no control of how it comes out of my mouth. Therefore, my written word is much closer to what I'm really trying to communicate.' -RJ

from the Legend- John Wooden-- 'There is a mystical law of nature that says the 3 things we crave most in life-- happiness, freedom, and peace of mind-- are always attained by giving them to someone else.'

The solution is knowledge, self-discipline and virtue. -CS

Sometimes I think that caring is a genetic defect. -RJ

Please consider this: it's quite possible that 99% of the aches & pains we run to the doctor for can be remedied with Intelligent Strength. (No drugs, no surgeries, no braces, no orthotics, no co-pays, no deductibles, no p/t, no adjustments) #OwnYourHealth -RJ

At My Back and Body Clinic you will be loved but never coddled! #RealStrengthIsTheAnswer -RJ

Let's just assume for a second that I know something that you don't know. But you believe what I know is something that you totally know as well. But you really don't. Now my task is to Not only teach you what I know, but also help you Un Learn what you have believed for a long time. -RJ

For all you really smart people this might just drive you crazy!! The longer you live there is a realization that there are more Questions in Life than Answers! -RJ

Fear, anxiety, & worry all make your physical condition WORSE & that includes PAIN. -RJ

1- get a very specific diagnosis from your doctor. 2- research your doctors solution carefully. 3- use drugs or a natural, organic solution & OWN your health.

Strength is for Service, not status. -RJ

The Strong take on the troubles of the troubled. -RJ

No matter what your doctor says, if you are on lifetime medications, you are not healthy. Own your Health. -RJ

That awesome moment when we realize that- no matter how miserable or poor or sick or broken we are- we can have an incredibly powerful, positive effect on another human being. - RJ Pause & think about that ☺

Strongman definition: 'One tough dude who crushes spikes, tears cards, lifts stones, snaps chains, shreds phonebooks, twists horseshoes, rolls frying pans, bends steel bars, and/or drives nails with one blow of his fist'...

One's Greatest Strength is in being created unique; One's Greatest Weakness is not believing it. -RJ Please pause & really Think about that-- Believing is quite Powerful!

Take control of YOUR health!

In this information age of so much mis-information, continue to seek TRUTH--- oh yes, you will learn some things!

The question is how long will it take you to sift through all the scams- training programs, supplements, diets, bad gyms, & the opinions of highly-edumacated folks who have no idea what they're talking about. ☻ -RJ

Minimal Exercise with Maximal Focus yields the Greatest Benefit! This 'truth' hit me yesterday after 40 years of 'working out' in all different types of training systems/philosophies. I can prove it! -RJ

If you ever run into any of my children, ask them at what age they learned about the word 'cumulative'... and then ask them if the Old Man was right or wrong... -RJ

Ya know Boys & Girls-- I've seen a lot & learned a lot over the years. Be careful who's advise you take-- just sayin'.

What if someday ALL the experts figured out that Butter is Good for You & the bread is bad?

If you want to be lean & healthy, Good Fats should make up over 1/2 of your caloric intake. It blows the this-sounds-logical mind to think that FAT DOESN'T make you FAT!!

C'mon people... it doesn't have to be this way. Just spoke with a woman who wanted help. She now weighs 296 pounds. Sweet lady who has 'tried' every ^(^&^*%*%&$(diet out there, has bought all the equipment & gym memberships. She wants me to teach her 'lifestyle'. No worries...

As I look at Conventional Wisdom, I'm reminded of how it is usually a trap and not really Wisdom at all! -RJ

Plz Pause & think about that---

Lotsa scams everywhere--- be Hungry4Truth!

Living in the Moment is radically impacted by one's Vision for the Future! -RJ

In this insanely helter-skelter world, it's Vitally important to take time to find a Quiet Place to Reflect & Pray & Capture your Vision and Dreams!!

The Peace & Excitement generated are Well Worth the time dis-connected from the grid!

Make your training FUN but never compromise POSITION! - RJ

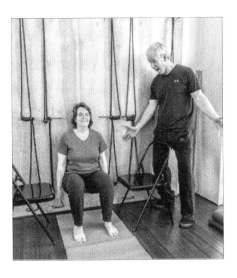

Basic Spike Bending using only Holy Rags! The 1st feat you train for when aspiring to be a StrongMan...

It was great fun watching a Young College Beach Muscled Stud fail to even crimp it in front of his school mates... then the GrandFatherly White-Haired one be able to crush it! LOL! Encouraging for me was not only the Young Man's respect but the overall Hunger for Truth that these College Kids had re Eating, Supplements, Training, Attitude... it was a great night...

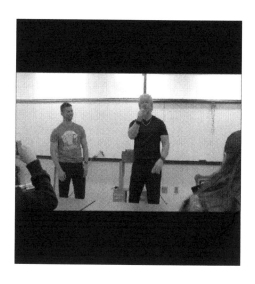

ATTITUDE BY CHARLES SWINDOLL

The longer I live, the more I realize the impact of attitude on life. Attitude, to me, is more important than facts. It is more important than the past, the education, the money, than circumstances, than failure, than successes, than what other people think or say or do. It is more important than appearance, giftedness or skill.

It will make or break a company... a church... a home. The remarkable thing is we have a choice everyday regarding the attitude we will embrace for that day.

We cannot change our past... we cannot change the fact that people will act in a certain way. We cannot change the inevitable.

The only thing we can do is play on the one string we have, and that is our attitude. I am convinced that life is 10% what happens to me and 90% of how I react to it.

And so it is with you... we are in charge of our Attitudes.

The End

Made in the USA
Middletown, DE
10 August 2019